D1596793

Mental Health Care in Crisis

EDITED BY ANNY BRACKX AND CATHERINE GRIMSHAW

PLUTO 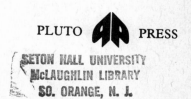 PRESS

First published 1989 by Pluto Publishing Ltd
11–21 Northdown Street
London N1 9BN

Distributed in the USA by Unwin Hyman Inc.
8 Winchester Place
Winchester MA 01890, USA

British Library Cataloguing in Publication Data
Brackx, Anny
    Mental health care in crisis
    1. Great Britain.   Mental health services
    I. Title II. Grimshaw, Catherine
    362.2'0941

ISBN 0-7453-0221-1

Contents

Contributors

Anny Brackx has worked as a journalist for 15 years. She now edits the mental health magazine *OPENMIND*.

Chris Bumstead is an occupational therapist. He has worked in Canada for several years and is now Co-ordinator of the Kirkdale Resource Centre.

Peter Campbell has been a regular recipient of NHS psychiatric services since 1967. Actively involved in self-advocacy he is also a member of Camden Mental Health Consortium (London), Secretary of Survivors Speak Out and a nursery nurse.

Alison Cobb is a Christian feminist and works in National MIND's Information Department. She has also been actively involved in promoting women's needs through the Women in MIND policy group.

Judy Donovan is Mental Health Tutor and Organizer for Yorkshire North District of the Workers' Educational Association.

Errol Francis works for the Afro-Caribbean Voluntary Health Association.

Catherine Grimshaw has worked in the Citizens Advice Bureau Service and National MIND for several years. She is currently employed at Rochdale and District MIND.

Dr Bob Grove has worked in therapeutic and similar communities for 15 years. He is an Assistant Director of the Richmond Fellowship.

Rick Hennelly is a project social worker based at North Derbyshire Mental Health Services Project, a part of Derbyshire County Council's Social Services Department.

Chris Holmes has written widely on housing issues. He is Housing Campaign worker for CHAR, the Campaign for Single Homeless People.

Andrew Milroy is the project manager of North Derbyshire Mental Health Services project. He is a social worker with a particular interest in mental health.

Naomi Narod was a picture researcher for 10 years. She now works as a volunteer for Amnesty International and National MIND.

Alison Norman was formerly Deputy Director of the Centre for Policy on Ageing, and currently works as a freelance researcher and writer. She has written several publications on mental illness and the rights of elderly people.

Harry Reid was born and brought up in Ireland but now lives and works in London. Involved in the campaign for the closure of psychiatric hospitals, he is a former Editor of the mental health magazine *Headlines* and a regular contributor to *OPENMIND*.

Dr Bob Sang was the first full-time advocacy worker in the UK. In the early 1980s he established the Advocacy Alliance project in several long-stay hospitals. Since then he has worked on the promotion and development of the concept of advocacy with many groups across the country.

Liz Sayce is a researcher at the National Unit for Psychiatric Research and Development, based at Lewisham hospital, London.

Ron Thomson has been involved in housing and mental health issues for ten years. He has personal experience of being homeless. Currently he is employed as General Manager for Newham Special Needs Housing Consortium, East London.

Preface

The big mental hospitals are closing down. In ten years most of them will have disappeared. Based on the principle that everybody has the right to lead an 'ordinary' life, people with mental health problems are to be integrated and 'cared for' in and by the community. Their basic needs for inexpensive and satisfactory housing, a decent income, something to do and the right kind of support, are neither startling nor extravagant. As the contributors to this book show, they form the bedrock of a care in the community policy. Yet without political commitment and proper funding such a policy remains, as always, admirable in theory but poor in practice.

The contributors also show that in order to be able to lead 'an ordinary life' in our society, people with mental health problems must acquire a sense of self-determination and control over their situation. This is difficult, for mental illness carries with it stigma and misunderstanding. In addition, the services on offer are frequently designed more for the convenience of those who run them rather than the requirements of those who use them. Altering attitudes can be as troublesome as securing the basic necessities for living outside the hospital. Nevertheless there are examples of changes for the better and they have been highlighted alongside the contributors' recommendations for action.

In short, this book is a siren call for community care to be resourced adequately and for mentally vulnerable people to be given a stake in a society which hitherto has largely ignored them. We want to influence those who are in a position to determine the shape of community care, whether it be politicians, planners, professionals or the neighbours next door.

Acknowledgement

The editors would like to thank Suzanne Cook and Paula Miller for typing the manuscript.

Introduction

ANNY BRACKX

This book was inspired by the voices of those people whose inability to cope with the pressures of a harshly competitive society or whose unconforming behaviour have forced them to spend time in psychiatric hospitals.

Both editors, and I am sure many of the contributors to this collection, are also indebted to a history of theorizing rooted essentially in the humanitarian liberalism of the late eighteenth century and culminating over one and a half centuries later in the UN's Universal Declaration of Human Rights.

In Britain the human rights of people suffering from mental health problems became the focus of attention from the late 1960s onward when stories about repressive regimes in mental hospitals and the scandalous conditions in these institutions became a regular news item. But it was Larry Gostin's contribution to the debate[1] and his tireless campaigning through MIND (the National Association for Mental Health) resulting in the Mental Health Act of 1983, which brought the whole issue into the public domain.

In a recent talk,[2] Gostin defines a human right as 'an entitlement due – legally or morally – to a human being'. So basic are these rights that 'they should be self-evident and permanent'. Yet despite these strong imperatives, he felt he had to spell out that 'mentally ill people, like all of us, have inalienable human rights.' The fact that this speech was delivered at an International Forum on Mental Health Law Reform held in Japan might well account for the explicitness.

Over 30,000 people diagnosed as having a psychiatric problem are detained involuntarily in Japanese hospitals. The International Commission of Jurists and the International

Commission of Health Professionals, in a 1985 report, drew attention to the abrogation of rights of those patients, particularly the lack of due process in dealing with involuntary detention, the absence of any review mechanism, and the profit motive in providing for the patients.[3]

Unfortunately Japan is not an exception; the rights of psychiatric patients are violated throughout the world and Britain's record is certainly not a clean one either. Part of the problem is that 'there is very little agreement particularly among lawyers and psychiatrists as to what these human rights are.'[4] The entitlement to humane, dignified and professional treatment may be an incontrovertible human right but others which seem equally obvious may well be less straightforward as they bring a host of professional and political interests into play. For example, the idea that people with mental health problems should have an opportunity to live an ordinary life, outside the social control often imposed by the psychiatric hospital, is to many as basic to their psychological survival as is good treatment, yet the concept is certainly not without its critics in psychiatric circles.

However, if human rights for people with mental health problems had been the focus of this book, a number of the authors would probably have found it a waste of time to contribute. Indeed, there is ample evidence in Britain that, even when some of those basic principles are enshrined in the law, this does not necessarily make it possible for people to use and enjoy them, nor does it guarantee that they will be respected. This is where liberal ideology falls short. It assumes that the law is an institution unfettered by the sordid imperfections of human nature. In a liberal democracy everyone is equal before the law, but as Peter Sedgwick points out, 'It is obvious that the pauper begging for pence outside the Ritz is less free than the cultivated upper classes who throng the tables inside.'[5] Legal confirmation may well be a prerequisite for further change, but until that more vigorous transformation in social and economic relations occurs which allows for a more equitable distribution of the nation's wealth, it is the well-educated, those with a regular income – individuals with a degree of status and power – who will be able to use the law most effectively.

We live in a society where market forces determine a great deal of our lives – a society that looks after those who look after themselves. Effective, self-reliant, productive behaviour is rewarded, dependence discouraged. Illness is a personal responsibility, old age a liability which has to be saved up for. The DHSS made this clear as long ago as 1976 in its document 'Priorities for Health and Personal Social Services in England'. It advises that 'The primary responsibility for his own health falls on the individual. The role of the health profession and of government is limited to ensuring that the public have access to such knowledge as is available about the importance of personal habit on health and at the very least no obstacles are placed in the way of those who decide to act on that knowledge.'⁶

Since 1979, when the Conservative government came to power, these policies have been consolidated. But is health really just a matter of individuals looking after themselves? The original Black Report, *Inequalities in Health*⁷ published in 1980 and the recent update, *The Health Divide*⁸ of 1987, show conclusive evidence that sickness and premature death are more common among poor people than among the better-off. Looking after yourself may well be a key factor in staying healthy, but a sizeable income seems to help matters along. Link these economic factors with ever more stringent cuts in public expenditure and an ideological climate which allows the government to erode the concept of entitlement to welfare benefits, and the merciless nature of laissez-faire capitalism becomes palpably obvious. Human rights, in this context, must indeed be hard to define and one of the most paradoxical areas with which to grapple.

Advocating 'care in the community' by closing what Sedgwick calls 'the warehouses of degradation', may not at first seem to fit in with this government's otherwise hard-nosed and business-like approach to social policy. Yet behind ministers' rhetoric of 'community care' and 'improving people's quality of life' lies very little action and one is forced to believe that what one is witnessing is simply a cost-cutting manoeuvre –

the transfer from a cost-intensive site to a low-cost site, from an administratively constructed site in which care is provided by specialized personnel under state auspices to sites located within the milieux of everyday life in which, to a greater or lesser extent, individuals (and their families) have, depending on their class positions, to make shift for themselves within the constraints of the subsistence existence available to those deemed "unemployable".[9]

Those 'milieux of everyday life' were first commended as an alternative to the isolated Victorian institutions by the Royal Commission on Mental Illness and Mental Deficiency (1954–7). Since then, the concept 'care in the community' seems to have taken on a life of its own, signifying 'good', as opposed to 'mental hospital' which for some years now has rightly been identified as stifling people's potentialities and autonomy. Nevertheless, community care is a highly ambiguous notion. It encourages romantic ideas of a cohesive caring society and hints at a number of supportive strategies which involve good neighbourly relations, a willing family and, above all, it assumes that local facilities and housing schemes are being developed at a rate commensurate to the running down of hospitals.

The truth of the matter is that there is no unified programme for transferring people from hospitals to places in the community. A few facts and figures quoted in MIND's evidence (July 1987) to Sir Roy Griffiths' View of Community Care indicate a decided lack of investment in such services. 'In 1984/5 there were 16,800 fewer people in psychiatric hospitals than in 1976/7. Local authorities must meet the costs to provide services for at least this number of people discharged from hospital. An estimate of the cost to local authorities over this period (Audit Commission) would be £240 million. The actual increase in local authority expenditure on mental health services for the same period has been £20 million.'

Mental health services have always scored very low on priorities of social services departments, but it is not just local authorities which are to blame for neglecting their most vulnerable citizens;

over the last decade, central government has increasingly put restrictions on extra spending through penalties and rate-capping. There are of course scattered examples of 'good practice' schemes: supported flats and housing complexes tailored to people's individual needs and situated in settings which enables them to use local facilities. Sadly, these initiatives are exceptional; they are 'the very "tip of the iceberg", and although useful in an experimental sense, there is no guarantee that public sector services will respond to tested "good" practice'.[10]

Without a drastic rethinking of resourcing and planning, it seems very likely that hospital closure strategies will amount to no more than what was witnessed during the closure of Banstead[11] in Surrey – the first major psychiatric hospital to shut down in the UK – where people were simply 'decanted' to various other institutions. In their review of housing and support in London for people leaving psychiatric care,[12] researchers Ada Kay and Charlie Legg recognize that there are fundamental financial problems underlying the implementations of a community care policy. However, they also stress that there are a number of other factors impeding satisfactory service delivery. Amongst these are administrative complexity and bureaucratic muddle, lack of coordination and inter-agency planning, structural and operational racism and poor user representation.

This statutory lethargy has already had far-reaching consequences encompassing a flourishing and by now notorious bed and breakfast trade which derives its profits from DHSS board and lodging payments, and a fast-developing market in private health care where very little enforceable quality control is in operation. According to *Laing's Review of Private Health Care*,[13] since the early 1980s, 'psychiatry has become one of the focal points of private health care.' They further point out that it is especially the sort of area 'where there are few existing public sector facilities and where there is no strong political pressure for self-sufficiency within health and local authorities that presents more fertile ground at present for contracted patient services than the acute sector.' Here too, growth is paid for by public funds.

More often than not, however, lack of local facilities just shifts the burden of care onto the family. The seat of wisdom, support and morality according to current Conservative ideology, it also happens to be the most cost-effective form of care in the community in terms of government spending. Already 'there are more women at home looking after disabled and elderly relatives than are looking after children.'[14] Conservatives call this type of care 'self-help'. As with 'community care' the government has been using the positive history surrounding the concept (in this case, taking a degree of control over one's life) as fancy wrapping for what amounts to neglect and a crude shirking of responsibilities.

In this impoverished interpretation, 'self-help' is 'making do', and far removed from its radical potential of people taking charge and organizing – at times enabled by sympathetic professionals – around their own needs and for a better deal in life. This action-orientated self-help has become known in mental health circles as self-advocacy. It aims to achieve maximum autonomy for people whose sense of self-worth, confidence and coping strategies have been knocked sideways through stress, breakdown and psychiatric institutionalization. In other words, self-advocacy is about empowering people to reclaim their place in the community as citizens. In their book *Advocacy and Empowerment*, Stephen Rose and Bruce Black explain that to enable people to play a part in the construction of their own life and destiny is half the battle won. Their approach was inspired by the principles of social philosopher Paolo Freire and developed over nearly a decade of working with former psychiatric patients in community settings in the US.

The move from passive consumer to more active producer signifies not only a shift in behavior in the social world, but a definite alteration in self-perception and self-judgment, a growing self-confidence restored to a person. Self-confidence gained through confrontation with an oppressive social reality and engagements in actions to transform this reality replace the self-contempt as characteristic of mental patient identity in a static world.[15]

As the self-advocacy movement gains momentum in this country so will the impact of users' views on the types of services that are being developed. Political and professional indifference will only be defeated through effective lobbying, pressurizing and exerting the necessary influence in decision-making bodies. Some authorities are already incorporating 'consumer consultation' and 'advocacy projects' within their planning and operational frameworks. But these are still only small dents in a system which has never had to consider patients' views. For the self-advocacy movement to grow in stature and influence it will have to persuade professionals to share their skills and expertise with the recipients of mental health care. Rooted in enlightened self-interest, such a partnership may well ensure that in future care in the community is better resourced and becomes an expression not only of people's various needs but also a reflection of their capabilities.

Notes

1. Larry Gostin, *A Human Condition Vols 1 and 2*, MIND 1975 and 1977.
2. Larry Gostin, Lecture at the International Forum on Mental Health Law Reform in Kyoto, Japan, 29–30 January 1987.
3. Chris Heginbotham, Editorial in *OPENMIND*, No. 29, October/November 1987.
4. Gostin, *A Human Condition*, 1987.
5. Peter Sedgwick, *Psycho Politics*, Pluto Press 1982, p. 176.
6. DHSS, *Priorities for Health and Personal Social Services in England*, HMSO 1976.
7. *Inequalities in Health*, Report of a Working Party, DHSS 1980.
8. Margaret Whitehead, *The Health Divide*, Health Education Council 1987.
9. Peter Barham, *Schizophrenia and Human Value*, Blackwell 1984, p. 178.
10. Nigel Malin, 'Community Care: Principles, Policy and Practice' in Nigel Malin, *Reassessing Community Care*, Croom Helm 1987, p. 4.
11. Harry Reid and Alban Wiseman, *When the Talking has to Stop*, MIND 1986.
12. Ada Kay and Charlie Legg, *Discharged to the Community. A Review of Housing and Support in London for People Leaving Psychiatric Care*, Good Practices in Mental Health 1986.

13. *Laing's Review of Private Health Care* 1987, Laing and Buisson Publications 1987.
14. M. Meacher quoted in Malin, *Reassessing Community Care*, p. 14.
15. Stephen M. Rose and Bruce L. Black, *Advocacy and Empowerment. Mental Health Care in the Community*, Routledge and Kegan Paul 1985, p. 101.

Part I
From the Horse's Mouth

1

Peter Campbell's Story

On Tuesday I woke up an hour before my alarm clock and wrote half a poem before going to work. I did a full day and worked an hour and three quarters unpaid overtime. The Christmas rush was coming and pressure was building up. On my way home a down-and-out approached me in Euston Station. I bought him food and spent two hours finding him somewhere for the night. By the time I reached home it was already late but I still managed to write three important letters before going to bed.

On Saturday I woke at dawn and left the house within an hour. I felt tremendous. Things had finally slotted into place and I was going to convert the 'natives' of the Upper Niger, equipped only with inspiration and a portable gramophone. Two hours later I tried to cross the Broadway opposite Hammersmith Odeon with my eyes closed. I laid my possessions outside the door to the church by the flyover and built a diagrammatic Calvary on the path. By mid-morning I was in custody, picked up by the police while standing in a bus garage, calling out about poisonous fumes in the earth. They locked me in a cell. I thought I was on the way down to Hades. Later they put me in a van and took me to a psychiatric hospital. I remember lying on the floor of a padded cell in my underclothes.

The above scenario is a distillation of events from 18 years as a user of psychiatric services. Whatever else it may reveal, I believe it illustrates a major feature of life for those diagnosed as mentally ill: loss of control. Loss of control, whether truly lost or merely removed by others, and the attempt to re-establish that control have been central elements in my life since the age of 18. My argument is that the psychiatric system, as currently established, does too little to help people retain control of their lives through periods of emotional distress and does far too much to frustrate their subsequent efforts to regain self-control. Whatever power I may now have over my life, I have, to a large extent, won in spite of rather than because of psychiatry.

Before describing the specific processes of psychiatry as I have experienced them, I wish to make two general points which concern the context within which the system operates. The first relates to the medical model, or more accurately to the assertion that the phenomena psychiatry deals in should be seen in terms of 'illness'. Whether we accept this approach or not, there can be no question that it provides the current framework for society's view of the subject and that the psychiatric profession must take responsibility. Psychiatry would see itself as the servant of society. Yet it is naive to suppose that a profession with such an individual and collective power does not form as well as reflect public attitudes. If we think of emotional distress as mental illness it is psychiatry that has seduced us so. And the pre-eminence of this concept does affect individual autonomy To live 18 years with a diagnosed illness is no incentive for a positive self-image. Illness is a one-way street, particularly when the experts toss the concept of cure out of the window and congratulate themselves on candour. The idea of illness, of illness that can never go away, is not a dynamic, liberating force. Illness creates victims. While we harbour thoughts of emotional distress as some kind of deadly plague, it is not unrealistic to expect that many so-called victims will lead limited, powerless and unfulfilling lives.

In the same way the feeling that the diagnosed mentally ill don't know what they are talking about, limits the scope of our lives. The concept of insight – perhaps lack of insight would be more appropriate from the psychiatric perspective – is one of the most powerful and insidious forces eroding our position as competent, creative individuals. If I am to be confined to a category of persons whose experience is devalued, status diminished and rational evidence dismissed, simply because at a certain time or times I lost contact with the consensus view of reality agreed on by my peers, then it is scarcely possible to expect that my control over my life will ever be more than severely circumscribed. If my experience is not valued I cannot be whole. It is in particular discouraging to speak to some psychiatric professionals and have my experience validated only as a particular and very sad blemish in an otherwise benign conception. This is no validation whatsoever. I am not the one regrettable bacillus in the sterile supplies room. My experience is shared and is relevant. It is not an interesting cul-de-sac. Tut-tutting and sympathetic frowns from those who are paid to intervene in my affairs merely confirms my powerlessness. They accept me as an individual pathology; they deny me as a cogent element of a social reality.

It is currently quite unclear whether those who work in the psychiatric system place a high priority on maximizing an individual's self-control during the process of breakdown. In this respect I find it significant that no psychiatric professional has ever advised me on how to cope with a breakdown beyond the blanket exhortation to keep on taking the drugs. My own experiences suggest that once I start to lose control again I am expected to admit powerlessness, hand myself over to the experts and count to 15,000. Such suspicions tend to be confirmed by the notably frosty reception my own ideas about my treatment receive from those who are attempting to process me back to in-patient status. It is clear to me that it is inconvenient to have to consider the integrity of the new admission too carefully during absorption into the psychiatric system. During admission, as at other times in the caring process, the system's needs dominate the individual's needs. This is bad enough as it stands. It is the more serious in view of the proposed shift to care in the community. A double dependency has been created. On one hand the users of existing services have been bred to accept dependency as a characteristic of relationships. On the other, the caring team have based their operations on this inequality. The danger is that community care will come to fulfil these expectations, those standard practices. Instead of dependency beyond the community we will simply be creating dependency within the community – small and beautiful institutions on the next street rather than large and ugly institutions ten miles up the road.

Whatever the intentions behind the system, the reality of current provision is clear enough. For most who experience severe mental distress there is only one destination – the psychiatric admission ward. Many of us – particularly those whose crisis occurs after hours of sunset – will find the journey there extremely unpleasant. I have found my GPs reluctant to visit me after dark, casualty departments where knowledge of psychiatry or psychiatric medications is peripheral, psychiatrists' secretaries who do their best to persuade me not to bother the doctor in times of acute need. In short a network of provisions designed to make it difficult for me to receive the help I may need and almost impossible to seek out the help I want.

If the admission ward met my needs I would endure the process of admission and the absence of choice as necessary evils. But it is becoming clear that for myself and for many others the admission ward is in no way a satisfactory environment in which to recover mental health. The existing system is not sufficiently sophisticated, those who operate it are not sensitive enough for whatever reasons to meet the real needs of the many individual people who are forced through it year after year. What is needed above all are alternatives to prevent so many people falling into the psychiatric system in the first place. Alternatives which do not rely on chemotherapy as a first choice response to crisis. Alternatives which address emotional distress as a problem of living and react to it more honestly than current psychiatric practices of 'patch up and put back on the road' allow. The impending closure of hospitals seems to have resulted in an obsession with the location of services. Character and quality of services is what really matters. Choice is essential. If provisions are to confront the real needs of people, it must first of all be accepted that people's needs are varied. It might even be worthwhile asking them what they want! What seems clear is that the same thing in different packages will be a golden opportunity tossed away.

In particular I object to the way in which power is stripped from me, the way that I am approached not as an individual but as a manic-depressive. It is not right that I should be casually drugged into unconsciousness on arrival in an admission ward. It is certainly wrong that I should receive treatment regardless of whether I arrive handcuffed to a policeman or walk in of my own accord and calmly ask for help. On two occasions I have been given so much medication that I fell asleep before admission formalities had even been completed. I have not yet been allowed to complete my own process of controlled breakdown without such ham-fisted interventions. While such practices remain common it is not possible to claim that psychiatry respects individual integrity or is much concerned with self-education or change.

The psychiatric system is founded on inequality. By and large, the user is at the bottom of the pile. I have been on wards which could not have functioned without the active help of in-patients. Yet when conflicts arose I have been told, 'What right have you to help with other patients? What would our union say?' I have met a few staff who clearly despise the 'mentally ill' and will openly abuse you. Their colleagues may agree in private that it is disgusting but they will always, in my experience, rally behind them when it matters. At times it is hard work not to believe that we are a separate branch of humanity.

Our unequal position is symbolized by the compulsory element in psychiatric care. I do not intend to argue either for or against the use of legal compulsion in treatment. But the fact of its existence has repercussions for all service users and these must be recognized. That an individual can be compelled to receive psychiatric treatment affects each in-patient regardless of whether his stay is formal or informal. It is hardly possible to be unaware that you are being cared for within a legal framework which allows for treatment against your will. Moreoever it is difficult for most in-patients long to remain ignorant of the belief – whether based on fact or legend – that the threat of legal compulsion may be used to coerce individuals to accept particular treatments. Whatever the justification for compulsion in care, an inevitable result must be the diminution, whether physical or psychological, of the in-patient's control over his or her life. The implications of compulsion, the contradiction which may exist between the concept of compulsion and the concept of care, would seem to have some part in explaining why many psychiatric patients look back on their time in hospital as punishment.

Our self-image is further damaged by the limited extent to which we can participate in our own treatment and in that of our companions on the ward. While the resources of the medication trolley are over-used, the human resources of those living and working in the psychiatric unit are consistently under-used. I have been on wards where experienced in-patients have almost had to 'book' time to speak to nursing staff. I believe that many nurses whose prime impulse is to care for those in their charge are working in an environment which prevents them from exercising their most important human skills. Certainly the potential of the in-patient to be a creative resource for the community of the ward is seldom realized. Patients do support one another. But staff attitudes to this are often ambiguous. I have seen the inside of numerous admission wards. With one exception none of them has provided structures which actively encouraged patients to be involved in one another's care. Most ward meetings studiously avoid 'emotional' areas and do more to confirm the powerlessness of the patient within a bureaucratic system than to encourage participation. I have a distinct suspicion that mental health workers in general don't like us to get too uppity.

I believe such an atmosphere belittles the standing of the so-called mentally ill. We are encouraged to be victims, to look vertically to experts for the solutions to problems they have defined, rather than to reach out for those around us who have a shared experience. We put down our positive capacities and assume instead the role of recipients of care. The concept of care in the community will remain pretty hollow unless it confronts this situation. The ethos within which we tackle our problems and are helped to do so is in reality damaging our chances of becoming partners in the community. If we are made to feel victims and powerless by methods of dispensing care, if we are made to appear inferior by the systems supporting us, it is more than optimistic to expect that relocating the service-points will miraculously end our isolation. It is what the psychiatric processes are doing to our status and our self-image that is important not where it is happening. I certainly support the move towards care in the community. But there are persistent and rooted obstacles to the so-called mentally ill becoming integrated into community life. The negative life-denying context in which we exist is not the sole responsibility of psychiatry. Even so it remains open to question whether the underlying psychiatric approach to its client group confronts or condones its isolation within the community.

Our restricted role in our own treatment is of fundamental importance. The 'good' patient is usually the one who does what he is told. In one hospital a charge nurse told me that I would not be welcome on his ward in future because I complained about the quality of care. The implication that I should shut up and be grateful is disturbing. Participation not passivity should be the bottom line. I don't see conclusive evidence that the psychiatric profession always knows what it is doing. Simply to keep repeating their sagacity in a loud voice does not mean that the experts are entering into dialogue.

At the crux of the dilemma is freedom of information. I don't believe a patient can be otherwise than powerless until he has reasonable access to information regarding his treatment. If there are choices of treatment then the patient should be made aware of them. I do not find it proper to suggest ECT as a treatment without explaining its limitations and side-effects and those of the alternative treatments which are available. It is wrong to suggest or to imply by omission that there is only one course of action when it is not really so. I have vivid memories of the trouble mental health workers used to take in the 1970s to suggest that psychotherapy was not available, impractical, too expensive. I also remember how jealously staff guarded information about medication. Patients like myself who knew something about the medications in the drug-trolley were treated with some suspicion. In general I have found psychiatrists prefer to tell you the absolute minimum about the drugs they have prescribed.

When I was put on Lithium Carbonate I was told that it did not have side-effects like other psychotropic drugs. It was four years before I was given a kidney and liver function test. Many of the side-effects of Lithium are precisely the same as psychotropic drugs – dryness of mouth, tremor, for example – and there are significant possibilities of further effects from long-term use. All of this I discovered from my own researches. As a result I was eventually able to weigh the pros and cons and make my own decision to remain on Lithium. But no thanks to the psychiatrists. The initial withholding of information, whatever its motive, denied me one chance of exercising adult responsibility.

I am not aware of any conclusive statistics that revealing the true effects of drugs to patients ensures they stop taking them. Many of us stop taking psychotropic drugs because they do not do for us the things we have been promised they will do. Playing up the positive effects and playing down the negative ones is a recipe for trouble. The whole approach to medication in psychiatry seems to be tinged with a belief that the 'mentally ill' are by definition incompetent and unable to be able to be adult even when returned to the community. Information is not volunteered and even when asked for directly, is given grudgingly and in inadequate form. As a result of not being told the possible side-effects of the depot (slow release) injection Depixol when I returned to the community, I suffered sporadic side-effects over a long period culminating in my collapsing with paralysis of the lower limbs in a North London street. This frightening experience could have been easily avoided. But to do so it would have been necessary for the system to recognize me as competent, adult and a partner in charge, not as a non-responsible recipient of care, biochemicals and established wisdoms.

Every system has its faults. I would more easily tolerate the iniquities of the process if the psychiatric system returned me bright-eyed and bushy-tailed among my contemporaries. But this it does not do. The percentage of readmissions is high. Moreover the diminished status we suffer while recovering from break-down is not made right once we re-enter society. Discrimination affects us on major and minor levels, in personal and public areas. Discrimination in employment is standard. There are many with psychiatric records who are forced to rinse their talents down the sink and take jobs far beneath their capabilities. I find it humiliating to have to lie in order to be in with a chance of work. To be advised to lie, to choose to do so and hereby admit a shame about my past which is not justified and which I in no way really feel, has demeaned me more than any other single event of my life outside hospital. I want a chance to be what I am and for that to be recognized as natural. Society is not only ignorant, it stuffs its ignorance down our throats as well.

My argument against the psychiatric system is not that it is uncaring. I have met individuals at all levels – nurses, social workers, psychiatrists – who were clearly caring people and cared for me. But psychiatry must surely be more than custody and care. By approaching my situation in terms of illness, by regarding me primarily as a recipient of care and treatment, the system has consistently underestimated my capacity to change and ignored the potential it may contain to assist that change. My desire to win my own control of the breakdown process and thereby to gain independence and integrity has not only been ignored, it has been thwarted. Throughout the last 19 years the major impression I have received is that I am a victim of some-thing nasty, not quite understandable, that will never really go away and which should not be talked about too openly in the company of strangers. In short I have been ill, am probably still considered to be ill and am in some sense or other certainly handicapped.

I can find little evidence that psychiatry challenges the nega-tive context within which the 'mentally ill' live. By losing control and having a nervous breakdown I seemed to have entered a particular dimension of existence which is defined by the fact of its inhabitants' inability to have control – of them-selves, their environment, their futures. The specific complaints I have made about the system's disempowering process are more worrying because they occur within an ethos that does not seem to challenge loss of power. Talk should be of creativity and change, not control and illness. Only then will the self-control I seek be a common object and not a by-product of protest.

2

Naomi Narod's Story

AN INTERVIEW BY DIANA SOUHAMI

Naomi and I have been friends since 1965. She has been ill seven times in the past 13 years with psychosis and depression. Doctors are uncertain in their diagnosis and she has no 'label'. Her most severe attack began in August 1980 and she was in hospital for over a year. She was treated with phenothiazines, semi-narcosis, Lithium, anti-depressants and ECT. Her marriage ended six weeks before she became ill and she has no relatives who are either able or prepared to help her.

She left hospital in October 1981 and went to Amadeus House, a Richmond Fellowship hostel in Ealing. She took part in the running of the house, had counselling sessions and gradually refound her confidence. Her recovery was slow – she was there nearly two years – but eventually she was well enough to reclaim much of her former life. She moved back into her flat, picked up on her social life and did voluntary work four days a week.

In February 1986 she had another acute psychotic attack and went into hospital again. She was there for six months. On both occasions when she was in hospital I and other of her friends worked out a rota of visitors, so that she saw one or other of us every day. Her consultants would not see us as we are not 'family' and our contact with the hospital was poor. The nurses seemed at best unapproachable and at worst hostile. And because of the system of appointing registrars for six-month stints, there was no one who truly knew her or her case. The DHSS spending allowance while she was an in-patient was £5.30 a week in 1981, and £7.65 in 1986, though she had her flat to maintain and was encouraged to go out in the evenings and weekends. She was involved in protracted legal dealings with her ex-husband who wished to discontinue paying her maintenance. Fortunately the court upheld Naomi's case and she now has a reasonably secure income.

The account which follows comes out of conversations recorded between us in March 1981, February 1983 and September 1986 – by which time she was living again in her flat, attending day-hospital, and slowly feeling her way, once more, into 'normal' life.

1981

Naomi: It's easier with physical illness, you're walking on crutches or you've an operation scar, but with mental illness it's something so intangible, your mind just goes. And there's a stigma about it. It's humiliating. On one level I want to broadcast to people, I've been ill, will you please accept me, on another level if I want a job ... I hope that if I come to terms with my illness other people might come to terms with it too. I don't think I have yet. It's been a great blow. I was doing so well ... I was due to go to America. I'd moved into this little flat in the Portobello Road, in London. I was gaining confidence and being independent and then August, always in August. I was dashed. My hopes were dashed. I think it's bloody unfair. I wouldn't wish anyone this illness, though having been through it I'm not afraid of anything else.

I had intimations that I was going to be ill – 'clunk-click' thought processes, word associations, my mind getting speedy. I phoned the hospital and my Lithium level was apparently low and they increased it over the phone. The consultant was away for six weeks after I arrived in hospital and I wasn't given enough Largactil. My body goes adrift if I don't have Largactil while I'm in this high psychotic state. The doctor said to me, 'I can see you're in distress' and I said 'distress ... my body needs chlorpromazine.'

I thought the Roebuck Pub was shining laser beams at us in the canteen to kill us. I thought the cash register when you buy a buttered bun or whatever said 'suicide' on it. I've also had the 'suicide squad' and the 'suicide pill'.

Those were my paranoid, disturbed thoughts. I thought that all the male members of the hospital had their right ears removed the way Van Gogh and Paul Getty's grandson had theirs removed. Total total madness I suppose.

I think I haven't inherited schizophrenia as such, I've inherited the predisposition to have schizophrenia or whatever it is. Maybe Ophelia had a predisposition towards madness, and because Hamlet was so cruel to her . . . The death of my father had a great effect on me, far more so than the death of my mother, though I have been ill five times in eight years – since my mother died in fact. I think it isn't just schizophrenia. I think the schizophrenic side was the hearing of voices, the hallucinations. My metabolism was eating me up. I didn't eat, I didn't sleep. My body felt bright red inside. There were people talking in my head. I could hear them and see them. I'd know that I was hallucinating, but they took over and I was out of control. I'm scared of losing control. I have a very low threshold of control against outside forces. I think that's where my vulnerability lies.

I'm fortunate to have been born with a certain amount of inner strength which has pulled me through. In the hospital I would say, 'Oh thanks to Depixol', but the nurses would say, 'It's not just Depixol Naomi, it's you. You've made the effort too.' And my friends have kept me on the go. They've been loyal to me when I've been low and when I've been high. They've told me that there is a world outside and that I will get better.

The following dialogue from this same conversation perhaps shows something of the all-round anguish of mental illness and how useful it might be if psychiatrists would find time to share what knowledge they have with those close to the patient:

D: When you were in one of those single rooms in the hospital, getting in and out of different clothes because you didn't know what to wear, your stockings round your ankles, wearing odd things in your hair, calling out that you wanted to die, you looked terrible, you seemed to be in such deep anguish such as I've never seen in another person. Do you remember quite what that suffering meant to you and was it as bad as it seemed to an outsider?

N: It was worse. I cried for nursing help and the nurses didn't come. I was told that I had to cry and be on my own the way a baby cries and is on her own. It was a pain in my head and I was screaming with agony and pain.

D: When you say a pain in your head do you mean a literal pain?

N: I mean a mental pain. They didn't tell me off, they just left me. I think it was necessary. It was part of the healing process. I had to let it out of my system.

D: That's like a sort of catharsis, whereas you looked absolutely dreadful. As if there was something organically wrong with you.

N: What, my yellow skin?

D: Your skin, your eyes popping out of your head, your inability to speak properly – the words tipping out one after another and sometimes not even words. Your identity seemed to be in tatters, but worst was the degree of anguish that seemed to go with it.

N: I shouldn't have been put in a single room so soon. I should have stayed in the dormitory with more supervision. I remember N. putting his arm around me and saying, 'You're not afraid of people any more, you don't think they're going to hurt you, do you Naomi?' And I was put in a room on my own which was freezing. And you and A. prepared the windows and got my slumberdown. I did prance naked before John M. because I thought my body looked good and I wanted to show him. I was quite ill, Diana.

D: Does it embarrass you that you behaved like that?

N: No, I don't feel embarrassed.

D: What about the locked ward? At the time of going into it

you were deeply offended and felt it to be like prison. You weren't allowed to see friends and I remember you saying that you thought all your friends were dead.

N: I suppose they're necessary, though they shouldn't be called locked wards. They should be called dorm four.

D: What led up to you being put in a locked ward?

N: I ate my own crap. A voice told me to kneel down by the loo and eat my own crap. And you found me and took me straight back to the hospital. I was compelled to do it. It was almost like someone hypnotizing me. Implanting thoughts in my head. My mother used to implant thoughts in my head. She used to say, 'Your father mustn't hear of any of this', when I was having an affair with that Persian boy. 'Your father mustn't know any of this.' And she would plant those thoughts hypnotically into my head. My head was like **an** Hieronymous Bosch painting. It was spilling over with implanted thoughts. And then I would have the opposite of that – my mind would go a complete blank. Horrible. Frightening. Not controlling your own destiny, but having someone control it for you.

D: Is that behind you now?

N: Yes. Yes. Yes.

Doctors tried everything to shift her psychosis and eventually after 12 days of semi-narcosis 'sleep-treatment', her mania subsided. Then followed a long period of depression, treatment with anti-depressants, ECT and Lithium, a suicide attempt and a second psychiatric opinion. When Naomi arrived at Amadeus House in October 1981 she was in a very fragile emotional state.

1983

Naomi: I've been at the Richmond Fellowship hostel for 15 months now. It's helped me tremendously. The staff come over as more humane, more caring. They give you time to listen to what you have to say on whatever you care to talk about. This term after-care is very important. When I was in hospital I was too ill to talk about my feelings. There were too many horrific things going on. They dish out the drugs, make sure you have your food, but that's all they can do and all you can do. But when you've recovered from the psychosis and you're shattered and you come to a half-way house it's a gradual building up of a person again.

I faithfully take Lithium although I was on it when I got ill in 1980. I didn't get ill last year, I don't know why. Maybe because I was at Amadeus in a secure situation where there weren't any pressures. I get tired and thirsty on Lithium and it slows me down but it's not too bad.

There's a lot of emphasis on practical things in the house. Some people don't even know how to make a cup of tea, they've been institutionalized for ten years or more, everything's been done for them, so it's a big thing that they can make a cup of tea for themselves. There's shopping, cooking lunch, cooking the evening meal with a partner. You share the chores. We have a catering group each week and we discuss menus – things like that. Then we have a community meeting on Monday. You have to attend and personal matters are brought up. I'm not able to talk at these large meetings. I find them too formal, too many people, but afterwards there's a small group meeting run by two staff members and I'm able to say things then.

I've been helped very much by having individual counselling for an hour a week. You learn to have insight. You try to make sense of what's happened to you up to this point. The sessions at times have been very harrowing. I'm conscious of benefiting from it, but not in any obvious way. For the first time I think I'm quite important and I'm concentrating on me. My own volition is coming into things. I don't seem to want a close relationship as desperately as I did before. My illness has changed me. When things change for you, your circumstances change, you're forced to change your outlook. I don't feel I've come down in any way but my values are different now. I don't think status is so important. I think I'm wiser.

I'm living a quieter sort of life. I want to get the pace right for when I leave the House. I want to leave well. Some people leave badly. You see if they knew how or why I got ill then obviously I would try and avoid whatever caused the thing, but since I don't know, I'm being very careful. I was humiliated in my illness and it looms over me.

I love coming back to my flat at weekends. It's as if I'm reclaiming it. I've got my bits and pieces there. My props. Most people at the hostel have nowhere to go and no money. When you're mentally ill you're penalized financially. I used desperately to make arrangements to see people over the weekend, but now I feel quite relaxed about it. I'm working two days a week at Amnesty International and enjoying it, also one day a week at another Richmond Fellowship hostel for people who have had drug problems. Both these are voluntary jobs. I don't want a paid job. It would make me feel pressured.

I'm determined to maintain support structures after I leave the hostel. I'd like to have psychotherapy. Dr. P. at the hospital is going to see me on a regular basis for therapy. I offered to pay to see her privately but she said 'I don't believe in paid medicine' and I said 'Oh good'. I'd like to talk about my low self-image, my family, my marriage. The last thing I want to talk about is my illness. I'm hoping to join a women's group locally and keep my good and faithful friends.

One of the things the hostel hopes to teach you is not to repeat the patterns of the past. If I'd gone straight back to my flat after the hospital I'd have stayed in bed and got depressed. I wouldn't have coped alone. It's given me higher standards. It's helped me get my confidence back. And counselling has helped me rethink my life. Life's worth living, albeit at a measured pace.

Apart from one bout of depression, which was treated with anti-depressants, Naomi stayed relatively well from the time she left the Richmond Fellowship hostel in autumn 1983 until February 1986. She slowly rebuilt her life and regained her confidence and independence. I asked her to describe how she managed to keep free from a hospital context during that time.

1986

Naomi: Probably the most crucial things were that I was on Lithium and having a life without pressures. I loved living in my flat alone. I liked doing things that I want to do, without having to refer to someone else the whole time. I used to buy flowers for the flat and cook nice things to eat. I enjoyed pottering around. I worked as a volunteer at Amnesty on Mondays and Tuesdays and at MIND on Wednesdays and Thursdays. Fridays I kept for myself.

My women's group was a focal point each Monday evening. They just let me weather it when I got depressed and didn't put on any pressure. It's a supportive group. And I had group therapy on Tuesday evenings at the Westminster Pastoral Foundation. It's a pretty high-powered group but you can get a lot from it. Other evenings I saw my friends. And I had a boyfriend. He helped me get back into the world. He helped me quite a bit.

My contact with the hospital was pretty minimal. I'd go along to out-patient appointments. I'd tell them that I was all right, I'd get a prescription for Lithium and I'd come home again.

I'd think about the terrifying things I'd been through in 1980 practically every day. But I felt extremely well. My life seemed to be in good order. People were pleased with the work I did. Then it became important for me to prove that I could get a paid job. There was a job going at MIND. It seemed the right organization for me to get a job with. And I wanted to come off Lithium. I wanted to be in control of what was going into my body rather than having that dictated to me. I felt confident enough and well enough to be able to say, 'Right, I'm going to come off this.' I did it not exactly with the approval of the psychiatrist, but he gave me permission . . . He said, 'Well, the Lithium is to protect you.' And my thought process was,

'Well, the Lithium is to protect the hospital.' But he was right. I didn't know. I didn't talk to enough people about coming off it. It was a terrible thing to have happened. It's the one thing I regret.

For four and a half months after stopping Lithium I was functioning extremely well. I lost weight, my skin was clear, I had more energy, I felt I could perceive things in a clearer, brighter way. I felt I could do almost anything. I didn't realize that I was going to embark on another psychotic illness. It was the same old thing again. And I wish I hadn't made that experiment. It wasn't worth it. Friends say I was more ill in 1980, but each bout of suffering is completely awful in itself. Quite, quite destructive. Destructive to me and to my relationships. Illness has changed me dramatically. Has taken my confidence, given me a low image of myself. But I'm glad I'm still here and I'm slowly rebuilding my life yet again after another devastating illness.

Naomi is now living once more in her flat, resuming her voluntary work, going out with her friends and attending her women's group. She separated from her boyfriend which caused her much sorrow. She has transferred to a smaller hospital in her own catchment area near where she lives. She goes there three days a week as a day-patient. She described how she felt about the two hospitals.

Naomi: I wouldn't give the Royal Free Hospital more than five out of ten. The staff seemed punishing. They'd tell you off if you did something wrong. When I first arrived I was in a terribly high state and unfortunately I vomited. I couldn't get to a sink in time. I was told, as if I'd been a naughty child, 'You clear that up.' I did, but I thought it was a shocking way to treat someone in the condition I was in. I didn't feel any warmth from the nurses at all. They could be more caring. I was so terribly frightened. I felt as if I was number 250 going through the system. I saw one nurse pulling a distressed patient by her legs down the corridor. And another nurse called to him, 'What are you doing?' And a friend of mine, a patient, killed himself. He'd been told to leave the hospital and he had nowhere to go. Some patients are just put into bed and breakfast places.

The nurses dole out the pills and hope you'll get better because it's less trouble for them. You couldn't have any one-to-one discussion. It was very lonely. And I felt not only estranged from myself but from the area. St Charles's is not only a smaller and more caring unit, but it's near where I live. It's true that I'm not so ill now but it does seem a better unit. I felt the Royal Free let me down badly when I left. They didn't seem too concerned about my future. I had an out-patient's appointment for a month away. That was all. Even though I'd been so terribly ill. The transition to my flat was too difficult for me. I'd asked to be visited at home by a community psychiatric nurse, but they didn't arrange it. I even wrote to them and asked, but I got no answer to my letter. I felt overlooked by them. I had to arrange it for myself through my GP.

At St Charles's there's a very good support structure. Each day we have an open group where we can discuss anything we like and there's a community meeting once a week attended by the doctors. We do a lot of practical things too: sewing, indoor gardening, cooking. I'm helping type up articles for the magazine which we're producing. There's yoga, move-ment, relaxation, pottery, art and so on. It's well organized. And I'm impressed by the calibre of the staff. They don't just concentrate on medical problems. They're kind and patient. Leaving is gradual. And when I do leave, the community nurse will visit me regularly in my flat. Everything's on a smaller, more human level. Though I do wonder were I to get critically ill again, what the standard of medical treatment would be.

I asked Naomi whether she felt privileged in having a reasonably acceptable income, a flat of her own and support structures of friends, counselling and voluntary work.

Naomi: It makes an enormous difference to me. I can have some dignity in my life. There's none if you have no money. There's one poor man who's a day-patient at St Charles's. He shambles in, sleeps where he can. If he finds a chair he'll sleep on it. He's always short of money. He lives in some hostel. His clothes are terrible. I say to him, 'Shaun, you should get a clothing grant' and he says he's not allowed one. I don't know what happens to people like Shaun. It's pitiful to see him. He has a dingy life. Last week there was a trip to Brighton. I said, 'Go on Shaun, it'll be a day out.' He said, 'But I don't have any pocket money.' Friends of the Hospital, a voluntary organization, gave him £2 and he had fish and chips on the beach and a nice day. But apart from private organizations like the Richmond Fellowship and voluntary bodies there's not much on offer for people. And there's still a great deal of misunderstanding about mental illness. When I was down the DHSS recently the man behind the counter was extremely rude to a claimant who was obviously very unwell. This isn't a caring society. It's everyone for themselves. You can't say to someone shuffling down the street carrying a million plastic bags and one on his head, 'Pull your socks up.' You can't say that to him. He's in his own mad world. Society penalizes you for being ill. You're given the bare minimum. Nothing more. It's absolutely crucial to have somewhere to live and something to do and not to be exploited. If you're worried about how you're going to pay the bills, or worried about how much you can spend on food, it can lead to break-down, I'm convinced of that.

Naomi has great courage. She battles with illness and tries to reclaim what is hers: her sanity, her dignity, her ordered life and her peace of mind. I asked her if she felt diminished by illness:

N: I felt that strongly when I was in Amnesty recently. People seemed so confident. I'm quite bright and jolly in the day hospital, but that's because I'm with people who are less well than I am. If you have a society of well and ambitious people then those who have been ill are going to feel left behind.

D: Are you afraid of life from now on?

N: Not at all.

D: Afraid of being ill?

N: We none of us like to be ill.

D: Afraid of dying?

N: I'm not afraid of dying.

D: Out of each of those three things which are you most afraid of?

N: Of being ill. It's such a devastating experience and it takes such time and effort to come through it.

D: Is that equivalent to saying you would rather be dead than suffer another bout of illness?

N: I can't bear the thought of having such an illness again and I probably wouldn't be able to remember that I can get through it.

D: But you can get through it.

N: I can say that now but at the time it's so overwhelming and eats me up so that I can see no let-up from it.

D: So you hate it now as much as you ever have.

N: Oh, absolutely. The whole experience has changed me. I don't take anything for granted now.

Part II
What Community?

3

Mental Health Education –
Developing a New Frame of Mind

JUDY DONOVAN

We are all educated in matters of mental health, and our most profound learning experiences will have preceded anything resembling formal mental health education.

Mine began in a Wisconsin farming village, populated by the children and grandchildren of the Scandinavian immigrants who settled the farmlands of the northern Midwest of the US. The experience of clearing land for farms and raising families on them made them copers and survivors, and their children, villages and institutions grew up to reflect and meet the needs of 'copers'. Mental health, if it existed as a concept, was a pragmatic one. The mark of sanity was the ability to manage, to survive – at its optimum, to contribute. Not all those early immigrant farmers, however, did manage: the endless hard work, coupled with the often intense isolation and loneliness must have contributed to what historians have considered as relatively high levels of suicide. There weren't many options to not managing, even temporarily.

In my village, during the 1940s and 1950s, there were more options, and life was not as demanding. Every community had, and tolerated, its 'non-copers' – the village drunk, the 'village idiot', the old. But not, on the whole the 'mentally ill'.

I do not, in fact, even remember hearing the term mental illness during my life in that village – I had only the vaguest notion of what depression meant, none at all of such things as schizophrenia or anorexia nervosa, and had never heard of a mental health centre. More importantly, I knew nothing of gradations of mental well-being: one either managed and was, by unspoken definition 'sane', or one went mad and went 'down-the-river' – over 200 miles, to the nearest state psychiatric hospital. As a child, I was afraid of being taken away to one of two places, by the Indians, to their nearby reservation, if I was bad, or to Mendota, the psychiatric hospital, if I couldn't manage.

For those who did go 'down-the-river' to Mendota, they either never returned, or they returned different to their former selves and were treated as different. To my knowledge, they didn't speak of their experiences. And the rest of us contained and protected as best we could our own corners of madness, lest our whole person become spoiled. We did not, as a community, know how to tolerate madness in ourselves or others; those who went away carried all our madness with them, enabling us to cope better. We made madness a thing apart, to be feared – the village cinema, featuring films with the occasional 'raving maniac', confirmed and gave shape to our own creation.

As an undergraduate in a Midwestern college, I discovered a theoretical framework to validate these experiences in a course called 'Abnormal Psychology'. As I prepared for my exam by memorizing the categories of illness falling under the two general headings of neurotic and psychotic disorder, I felt – rather than perceived – familiarity. A neurotic disorder meant, in essence, impaired coping ability; a psychotic disorder implied the breakdown of normal coping powers.

The loss of normal coping powers took with it status, personal power and dignity, as confirmed by our class visit to the local state psychiatric hospital. Here, specimens of various learned categories were duly paraded across a small stage and were asked questions designed to elicit appropriately symptomatic responses. I saw mania, depression, schizophrenia – labelled and in the flesh. (As a class, we were warned against responding to any requests by off-stage patients to post letters; they might be addressed to local politicians, even to a senator or the Governor, and would only cause annoyance and bother.)

Later that year I became a volunteer visitor at the same hospital. I visited locked wards, talked to nurses and the occasional doctor but, most important, I began my first prolonged acquaintance with someone diagnosed as mentally ill. Through

Tony, a 17-year-old 'psychopath', I began to unlearn, re-learn and to learn about mental illness and mentally ill people. I took, unknowingly, my first real steps towards acknowledging and understanding 'corners of madness' in myself and others, and began a gradual redefinition of mental health in its broadest terms.

Now, in the North of England, I am professionally involved in mental health education at a time when changes in mental health care are inviting a re-examination of thinking and feeling in mental health. Those involved in the process will bring to it, as I do, their own profound accumulation of learning.

The business of defining and discussing mental health education in its broadest and most positive terms is not the purpose of this article. Rather, I wish to concentrate on the enabling role of education in specific regard to present policies of 'care in the community' for large numbers of mentally vulnerable people. How can education help individuals and communities to extend their boundaries to encompass those mentally vulnerable members in ways which are beneficial and satisfying to all its members?

In exploring this question I draw primarily on eight years of experience and experiments in my present community in North Yorkshire, but my exploration has drawn me again and again back to my first community in rural Midwest America. Perhaps because it was long ago and far away, some things about that community's attitudes towards mental illness and mentally ill people have emerged for me as touchstones in my present thinking about mental health education in a community which is not mine by birth. And sometimes, with ears attentive to those early voices, including my own, I hear more clearly the voices of people in my present community.

1. In my village, a working definition of mental health/ill health which had developed in response to the demands imposed by survival in that particular community, became a normative definition.

2. Community institutions embody and maintain received norms and protect the community from threatening deviations.

3. Other institutions develop to manage 'differentness' by containment and separation, and new idioms develop to translate this management into popular shorthand.

4. Some forms of deviation are tolerated and contained within the community through assigned roles.

5. Identifying and separating 'mad' people from the rest of the community serves a function: such people can carry a burden of madness greater than their own. In such a situation, 'sane' people have a vested interest in maintaining madness.

6. 'Sane' people, denying and denied their own madness, will displace their own fears and anxieties on larger-than-life madmen. The more stringent the community taboos, the larger the figures of madness. These figures, in turn, increase fears.

7. Face-to-face meetings with people known to have experienced mental illness become increasingly characterized by unease and awkwardness.

8. Ignorance is a vacuum to be filled by fear, mystification and stigma.

9. Communities which strip their mentally vulnerable members of status, power and personal dignity come to see such losses as the effects of illness and as evidence of further, irremediable differentness.

10. Conceptual models of illness can be self-actualizing and can serve the vested interests of the 'sane'.

11. Where madness is perceived as 'infecting' the whole person, even ordinary requests and behaviour can be interpreted as symptomatic of illness and mad people have little opportunity to investigate their sanity.

12. Any significant personal contact between a 'sane' and a 'mad' person must throw into question the assumptions that prop up such conceptions – not because mental ill health is a fiction, but because concepts and definitions which have been subverted into tools for the effective

management of mental aberration, belie the true nature of the experience.

If there were a number 13, it would have to be in the form of a question: can education help to develop the informed awareness which changes even attitudes and behaviour so deeply invested with a sense of personal and community identity?

One answer comes from a study of a comprehensive mental health education programme carried out in 1951 in a small Canadian prairie town not unlike my own village.

The study was designed to investigate to what extent and in what directions attitudes towards mental illness are changed by an intensive educational programme ... The most telling point of this study was that, despite the use of competent educators using the best available educational material, this attempt to enhance tolerance and understanding of mental health problems was an outstanding failure. In fact, in trying to modify community attitudes to mental health the programme only succeeded in provoking anxiety and open hostility on the part of the local population. By attempting to change existing attitudes towards mental illness, the educators would appear to have undermined the community's existing ways of dealing with their feelings about mental illness. By questioning these mechanisms, whereby community solidarity and equilibrium were preserved in the face of mental illness, the team managed only to destroy the community's faith in the effectiveness of its own defences.[1]

The findings of other experiments, however, are less conclusive; another study, ten years later in an urban environment, indicated much more informed and positive attitudes towards mental illness, leading the authors of the study to suggest that there may have been a growth in the public's awareness of the nature of mental illness over the past ten years.[2] Certainly attitudes do change, but the relevant question here is, can education facilitate positive changes in attitudes?

It is interesting to look at a very recent survey carried out in a North Yorkshire comprehensive school (it is worth noting that the head teacher of the first school contacted refused to co-operate in the survey. 'I do not wish to subject my children to such material.') On the basis of 73 questionnaires completed by a group of mixed-ability boys and girls between the ages of 14 and 16, the authors of the survey felt they 'had no sweeping hypothesis to prove or disprove', but the data indicates a relatively high level of acquaintance with current psychiatric language – with varying degrees of real understanding – and, more significantly, a low incidence of unrealistic ideas about psychiatric patients and violence, a desire on the part of 64 per cent to know more about mental health/ill health, and a clear majority (71 per cent) thinking it was a good idea for the mentally ill person to live in the community. When that 'good idea', however, was translated into, 'Would it worry you if a group home was established next door to your home?', 51 per cent responded affirmatively, and a larger number (66 per cent) thought that their parents would worry. It would be interesting to explore the interplay between the pupils' desire 'to know more', their discrepancy between stated belief and feeling, and the 'worry' imputed to parents, only partially owned by the young people themselves. [3]

Though we do not know what their parents' responses might have been, such imagined responses might be compared to the responses of residents in another Yorkshire community when informed of plans to accommodate mentally ill adults in their neighbourhoods.

In 1984, in response to the local Mental Health Association's application for planning permission to convert a residence into a six-person hostel, most people on the street signed a petition against the proposal. They objected on two grounds: property values would go down, and children would be endangered. Though planning permission was eventually granted, the City Council criticized the Association for not establishing better relations with the local community (only three neighbours had been contacted), and the local press headlined their account of the proceedings, 'Crisis Seen in After-Care'. [4]

In fact, the Association was 'gazumped' and they later repeated the exercise in another neighbourhood, this time writing, telephoning or visiting about 65 households in a process of consultation and information-giving. In the end, two people objected, suggesting that it was unfair to put such people on a busy road. Those involved in the canvassing decided against a public meeting, feeling that this might stimulate rather than allay anxiety, and decided on personal contact as the best way of providing information, reassurance and the opportunity for consultation.

The Health District, in its bid to house approximately 14 men on a quiet residential street, wrote to everyone in the street at the same time as the decision to purchase was reported in the local press. The letter invited contact with the Senior Nurse Manager responsible for providing information, discussing problems and generally in engendering good relationships in the neighbourhood. After some initial anxiety and fear, the response was considered, overall, a favourable one. The main worry that was expressed concerned increased traffic in a cul-de-sac, although one woman was fearful for the safety of her young adult daughter (fear of physical and sexual violence). Two years on from 'Crisis Seen in After-Care', the same local paper, reporting that 'the District Health Authority is going down the much misunderstood road of community care', headlined its account: 'Mental "Stigma" to End'.[5] One MIND worker involved in establishing the group homes feels that, in view of the relatively good existing relationships, the kind of education which is needed is of a practical kind, in looking at how people can be 'good neighbours'.

No single factor accounts for these differences in response (for example the first neighbourhood cited was of a more homogeneous nature than the second, which had within it a wide variety of accommodation).

The experiences outlined above seem pretty clearly to indicate that anxiety is often the anxiety of 'not knowing', and that education in the form of straightforward information and reassurance might dispel it and allow more positive attitudes to emerge.

This is not, however, always the case (as indicated in the findings of the Canadian study); and in view of the initial anxiety in all of these accounts, the school-children were probably right about their parents' responses, even though the same parents might, like the children, have also supported the general idea of community care. The discrepancy between belief in principle and ambivalent feeling seems a key area for exploration in mental health education – that at the point of reconciliation of what we think with what we feel the kind of profound learning that leads to changed attitudes and behaviour can occur. The findings of the Canadian study are, in some ways, deeply at odds with the belief of Carl Rogers, that classroom climates conducive to significant changes in individual and group attitudes can be achieved. When such a climate is present, he maintains that 'learning of a different quality, proceeding at a different pace, with a greater degree of pervasiveness, occurs ... The student is on his way, sometimes excitedly, sometimes reluctantly, to becoming a learning, changing being.'[6]

My own experiences as student, teacher and organizer suggest that learning environments conducive to the positive exploration of attitudes in mental health can be created. In groups specifically designed to explore attitudes towards mental illness and mentally ill people, I try to create an environment within which underlying contradictions between feelings and beliefs can be safely explored. One useful way of 'giving permission' for such exploration is to begin with publicly-owned messages: a brainstorming of popular idioms for mental illness ('nutty', 'loony', 'crackers', 'round the twist', etc.) will very quickly lead from the release afforded by laughter (and laughter is usual) to critical examination.

Occasionally I use direct arousal of fear, contained within the safety of the classroom space, as a step towards dispelling fear and trying to move nearer a more realistic understanding of the experience of living with illness. I recall working with a group of educationalists wishing to pick up some ideas about mental health education. It seemed important that they should also experience something of that process themselves; and so I planned to begin with a discussion of the film *Halloween*, which had appeared on television only the night before. The film was classic in design: on Halloween, when strange and eerie disguises confuse identities and people are not as they seem, a psychopathic 'maniac' escapes from the local asylum and menaces a teenage girl. As it happened, no one had seen the film but, with the barest suggestion of plot from me, they quickly and accurately unfolded the story of a film they had never seen – derisively in part, but also acknowledging the power of the shared scenario they all carried in their heads.

Following on, one woman in the group spoke of her fear of walking alone at night since a number of young men, ex-psychiatric patients, had to come and live on her estate without – she felt – adequate support and supervision. Her account offered a number of lines of enquiry for herself and the group, all of them in some way dealing with the separating of rational and irrational fear. Such a group might usefully have continued this exploration with the aid of one of several recent television documentaries on 'community care': the power of film and television to exploit is equally a power to educate. Additional aids to exploration of attitudes in mental health are the education packs devised by CSV/MIND and ESCATA.[7]

Sometimes we can learn by confronting deeply-held fears directly, but a far more effective and natural way of learning is to acknowledge the reality that contradicts the fear. In plain words, we need to get to know and learn from the people who have first-hand experience of mental illness. And I believe that a formal learning environment can be an ideal place for that to happen.

I rediscovered this simple truth not quite accidentally, but incidentally, even though I had long since experienced it myself.

A few years ago I was involved in organizing a short course of open meetings for the general public, broadly designed to develop a more informed awareness of mental health issues; we were to consider specific kinds of mental health problems and both self-help and professional help for them. The six meetings were intended as a 'taster' from which we hoped to gather ideas for future courses with more particular focus. The format was similar for each meeting – a brief introductory session, essentially informative and usually in the form of a panel followed by small group discussion and plenary. The course was entitled 'Mental Health Problems' and the poster, distributed widely throughout the community, read: 'Have you ever wished you were better informed ... about mental health problems?' We chose the title carefully, wishing to avoid the total separation of mental well-being and ill-health and to stress the educational nature of the exercise. But we wondered and worried about our attempt to address a 'general public', knowing that we would be met by individuals with individual concerns and preconceptions. Would people come looking for personal advice? Could we provide for mental health professionals as well as the public? Would we raise expectations which couldn't be met in our community? What would happen in the discussion groups? Would anyone come?

In the end, people did come – over 70 people to the first meeting – and our wide advertising had paid off: no single interest seemed to dominate the group, and we had successfully attracted many people who were not otherwise involved in adult education. At that first meeting a clinical psychologist introduced the concept of mental health/illness as a continuum of difference, rather than a difference in kind, and described in specific and practical terms the ways in which we all change our positions along that line for shorter or longer periods. She provided facts and concepts, but most important of all her remarks provided a framework within which to explore our own questions in small groups.

And it was in those small groups where people learned – not simply from talking and listening, but from the uneasy confrontation of preconceptions about mental illness by the reality of the people who experienced it. I recall in one of the groups listening to the sharing of views between an older and a younger woman and observing the jolt of disturbed assumptions when, in the course of the conversation, the younger woman mentioned that she was presently resident in a psychiatric hospital and had joined some of her fellows to come to this meeting. Again and again, people learned from one another about the anxieties of parenting an anorexic daughter, the depression that so often accompanies enforced unemployment, the problems of facing neighbours after a period of hospitalization for mental illness, the discomfort of meeting friends who had been hospitalized for mental illness, the experience of living with schizophrenia.

The invitation to explore mental health/illness as a continuum offered no answers, but it disallowed the identity labels which so many students in mental health classes wear ('professional health worker', 'patient', 'interested observer') and encouraged the formulation of the real questions hidden by labels and categories. The title and venue of the class (college premises) provided a maximum of information-control; self-disclosure, when it happened, was spontaneous and relevant to learning.

At this time several people requested more specific information on depression; so shortly after these meetings we organized an open meeting entitled 'Depression – What's It About?' On the night, over 100 people more than filled the large room, and we repeated the exercise two weeks later, for 40 people. A panel composed of a GP, a psychiatrist, a young man recently recovered from a depressive illness and a social worker introduced the topic, followed by questions and discussion in the group. Not surprisingly, most of the early questions were directed to the psychiatrist as the accepted authority on such matters. As people became more easy in such a large group, they directed more and more of their questions and comments to the young man, who spoke with the authority of his experience. In turn, people shifted from the young man to one another, and the large meeting began to feel like a much smaller group as a wide range of people addressed the subject and experience of depression from a variety of perspectives. That meeting provided the impulse of a self-help group and a more formal course examining a variety of mental health problems often associated with particular times in people's lives.

It is perhaps too idealistic to imagine a programme of mental health education consistently attentive to the contributions of all its members, a forum consistently empowered and directed by real needs and experiences and leading towards a more informed acceptance of difference. But as an ideal, it seems worth pursuing – in tenants' associations, in industry, in churches, in adult education organizations, in schools and in small neighbourhoods where shopkeepers, residents and workers of all kinds can look at mental health issues relevant to their own community.

Recently several people involved in mental health education of varying kinds within our community have begun to meet as a group, hoping more successfully to identify and meet local mental health education needs. The meetings have also become a forum for ourselves – a learning space where we can question and explore the assumptions which inform our education policies and initiatives.

At the 'drawing-board' stage is another project, initiated by the Workers' Educational Association. As a part of an established adult education programme for people with mental health problems, we hope to organize a class in basic science at a local comprehensive school, recruiting students from the large numbers of ex-psychiatric patients living in sheltered accommodation in the immediate neighbourhood. Students at the school would be invited to assist the tutor by helping individuals in the class with a variety of science experiments. In return for their voluntary service, the young people would themselves attend mental health seminars designed to develop more positive and helpful attitudes towards mentally ill people. Central to this proposal would be the opportunity for young people to experience mentally ill adults as people with enquiring minds, capable of learning and developing new interests.

This kind of learning is liberation from fear and leads to empowerment – not simply to be more personally accepting, but power to modify and change existing institutions and policies. Policy-makers can impel proximity of residence as more people with mental health problems live in our communities – but we can impel policy-makers to assist us in making community care work in a way that all of us are better served.

Before writing this article I talked to quite a few people in my community about their ideas and experiences; among them were a group of people in a residential psychiatric unit which has since moved 'into the community'.

They had so many ideas, that the effect was a bit like a brainstorming session; the much abbreviated gist went something like this:

K: Attitudes are worst when it comes to employment – if you tell the truth, there's no chance. But it's a look on the face, rather than anything said.

A: Yes, particularly in the 'caring' professions!

G: MIND should have a positive discrimination policy for employing ex-psychiatric patients.

A: Employers need to understand the problems of mental illness.

G: The ignorance of people who don't know about mental illness! You tell them – and the relationship is different.

P: Well, I find that with people who knew me before I was ill, it's OK ... With strangers it's not.

K: It's something about not being able to control the information given about us too.

T: That kind of information should come from us – from people who have suffered illness.

G: They have to meet and know people who have been ill – education involves knowing!

A: But money needs going into this education – just like money goes into things like community relations projects.

K: Money for something like a film made by psychiatric patients.

T: Yes, that's part of it – mobilizing the strengths and skills of ex-psychiatric patients as a group is part of mental health education.

G: Pathetic ... spineless ... hopeless ... dependent ... that's the picture people have of us.

O: (angry) You know – all this, living here ... it's all make-believe. It's not like going back to live with your neighbours.

P: Well, I'm treated as ordinary in my village.

S: (quick retort) ... But what is ordinary?

Notes
1. Maxwell Jones, *Social Psychiatry in Practice*, Penguin 1968, pp. 48–9.
2. Ibid., p. 57.
3. D. Wright, J. Foster and J. Beck, 'Mental Illness – How School Children See It', *Nursing Times*, 17 September 1986.
4. 'Crisis Seen in After-Care', *Yorkshire Evening Press*, 24 August 1984.
5. 'Mental "Stigma" to End', *Yorkshire Evening Press*, 10 July 1986.
6. Carl Rogers, *Freedom to Learn*, Charles E. Merrill Publishing International (USA) 1969, p. 115.
7. *INSIGHT: Mental Illness in Perspective*, CSV/MIND 1984. *LIFE-STYLES for People who have a Mental Illness*, ESCATA 1984.

4

Women's Needs

ALISON COBB WITH JAN WALLCROFT

Women Who Care

Community care as it exists rests on the unpaid or low-paid labour of women. There is no sign that the government's plans for the future will lessen this load; in fact it is more likely to be increased, with the closure of mental hospitals, while inadequate finance is being provided for alternative local mental health care.

The expectation that women will pick up the pieces as the big institutions are phased out, is in keeping not only with women's traditional social role, but with economic policy which builds on and reinforces these traditions whenever successive governments find it useful. When women's presence in the workforce was needed during the wars, they were encouraged to enter jobs which previously had been seen as exclusively masculine. Afterwards they were expected to return to the home to allow men to take back their jobs. The back to the home tradition was achieved by intensive propaganda campaigns and pseudo-scientific theories 'proving' that women were not psychologically cut out to work outside the home, and that their 'natural' function was to care for their children, their men and their sick or elderly relatives.

In societies dominated by market forces women have come to represent a flexible pool of labour which has various uses: women's work can replace men's during war, supplement it during periods of expansion, and substitute for expensive unionized labour during recession to keep wages low. Today, though most women expect to spend much of their lives doing paid work, the type of jobs in which women are typically concentrated are part-time, low-paid service work, clerical work, and work in industries such as clothing which has been traditionally largely female. Because so many women have to work part-time they are less likely to be in a union. Unions however have often failed to protect the jobs of their women workers because of the ideology that women only work for a few extras and do not really need the money; that men earn a 'family wage' which is meant to support their women; and because of the fear that if women's pay and status is raised, men's will correspondingly be lowered. Women's paid work, therefore, tends to be insecure and it is relatively easy for them to be displaced from their jobs when the economy is under pressure, as it is now.

Women's sense of responsibility is used against them to undermine their position as workers – nurses are consistently underpaid and unable to take strong industrial action because of fear of harming their patients. Similarly women with children, elderly or mentally distressed relatives have little choice but to take on the whole burden of care when services are cut back, and to leave their jobs or to take low-paid jobs such as cleaning or homework which fit in with their caring duties. This makes good economic sense for the present government – while industry is allowed to collapse and work is scarce, many women can be removed from employment without adding to the unemployment statistics, thus making it easier to reduce public expenditure still further.

It's Enough to Make You Mad ...

Care-giving is central both to women's role and women's mental distress. A girl grows up learning to be attentive to the wishes and reactions of others. She develops what Luise Eichenbaum and Susie Orbach call 'emotional antennae' which anticipate other people's needs.[1]

As an adult she looks after the emotional needs of others, mainly at home, but often also at work and other social contexts. She lives a contradiction; stereotypical femininity does

not consist of adult traits, it is characterized by weakness,
dependency and deference. Yet a woman is expected to mother
all her family, without anyone to mother her. Because she has
learned to defer to others' needs she does not value herself
except in relation to those she nurtures (the 'empty nest' of
middle life is potentially liberating but very often is not in fact).
Because she does not value herself, she does not recognize her
own needs or, if she does, she feels she has no right to be
nurtured. While she takes responsibility for the emotional well-
being of those around her, her own neediness stays hidden.

'I somehow felt it was my fault when my husband stayed out
all night. I even had the feeling he was justified whenever he hit
me – after all I was jealous' said one woman reflecting on her
breakdown. And another, 'I married, had children and devoted
myself to being a good wife and mother, suppressing my own
needs and regarding my moods of depression and lethargy as
selfishness and laziness.'[2] A counselling service in Leeds finds
that some women feel self-help groups to be yet another burden
rather than a support because taking time out for themselves
goes against all they have learned.[3]

Black women are in addition subjected to attitudes based on
racist stereotypes, either denigrating or idealizing. For example
there is the 'docile, passive Asian woman' or the 'dominating
Afro-Caribbean woman'. And in terms of caring roles there is
the capable mother, lynchpin of a supportive and ever present
family network, immigration laws notwithstanding.

Living in a society which considers you either do not need,
or have no right to support is hardly conducive to mental
health.

'. . . but it's safer just to break down and cry'[4]

Twice as many women as men are treated for depression. Depression is an outcome of powerlessness. People who are in
distressing or defeating circumstances which they cannot
change, are vulnerable to it. One of the most important factors
in preventing depression is having someone to confide in – a

partner or close friend.[5] Child care, or caring for other dependants, puts limits on a woman's autonomy as well as her access
to friends; depression has been called an occupational hazard
of motherhood.[6]

Anorexia and other eating problems can be seen as a last-
ditch attempt of a woman to make an autonomous stance, in
the only way open to her, by controlling her food intake and
the size of her body. In the most extreme conditions of powerlessness and isolation – in the psychiatric wing of Holloway
prison – women have in their desperation mutilated or killed
themselves.

Doctors treat anxiety and depression – the symptoms of
powerlessness – with prescriptions of tranquillizers and anti-
depressants. In medicalizing these responses to life and in its
approach to the treatment of women generally, psychiatry
reinforces the stereotypes of women's role and compounds the
difficulties they create. For example, psychiatric definitions of
health for women, identified in 1970, include being 'more
submissive, less independent, less adventurous, more easily
influenced, less aggressive, less competitive, more excitable in
minor crises, having their feelings more easily hurt.'[7] These
contrast with a definition of adult mental health which coincides
with the masculine stereotype. Thus, strength in a woman can
be seen as insanity.

Furthermore, at a time when self-esteem is at its lowest – and
confidence is perhaps one of the most precious things a woman
needs to regain – she is placed in a relationship with her doctor
which for her often proves an infantilizing experience and
undermines the possibility of her self-image being redeemed. As
one woman said of her treatment in hospital for anorexia, 'I was
treated like a child who didn't know my own mind and needed
the psychiatrist to prescribe what was best for me. Now I feel
that much of what I went through had no effect on my eventual
recovery.'[8]

Too often cultural factors are used to explain away complex
life situations,[9] so an understanding of a particular culture in
general terms does not necessarily lead to appropriate help in a

specific situation. Racist assumptions on the part of health service staff, 'I'm sure the extended family will support her', 'These people never go to clinics', 'They don't talk about their feelings'[10] and the belief that black people cannot utilize talking treatments, result in black women being doubly disadvantaged when it comes to getting real help.

Assessment of a woman's recovery may be made in terms of her ability to perform household tasks and rehabilitation may consist of being offered a very limited range of activities in line with stereotypes of women's work.[11] Access to mental health services is limited for women by the lack of child-care provision at day-centres and other facilities. At one and the same time, women are scapegoated and relied upon by psychiatry, as mothers are blamed for the outcome of their children's development and yet are expected to be at the frontline of community care.

Doing it for Love

The statistics show informal carers to be an 'invisible welfare state'. Some one and a quarter million people are estimated to be caring for dependent relatives.[12] Of these 75 to 85 per cent are women.[13] In one sample survey 13 per cent of the women were caring for a sick or elderly relative.[14] A door-to-door survey in the North of England found more such carers than mothers of children under 16.[15] A survey in the Brighton area gives a picture of the typical carer as 'a woman, often older, with financial difficulties, often with children and probably also with a male partner to look after.'[16] Many have paid jobs.

Caring is costly not just financially, but also in terms of physical and emotional strain. The enormity of the choice (where it exists) whether or not to take on the main responsibility for the care of a dependent person is staggering. The consequences for the nature and quality of life of carer and cared-for and the relationship between them are far-reaching. A study of the recipients of Crossroads Support services found that most carers had undertaken the role for more than three years and a third had done so for at least ten years.[17] Few had time or energy for social interests outside the home. Less than one in ten had been on holiday in the previous two years. A study of key relatives of people with mental problems found 'a marked tendency for female members of the family to take the weight of responsibility, both practically and emotionally'.[18] Most respondents found their marriages affected – either significantly worse or noticeably better.

Both these studies point to the difficulty carers can have asking for help. For women this is reinforced by socialization into the caring role – we expect to do it because it is our job. If a woman has been coping for some time, the need for outside help can be experienced as failure. The dependent person may reject other helpers and emotionally manipulate the carer. People who know they are seen as strong and competent may be reluctant to expose their feelings of anxiety or depression. Where help is sought, and support services do exist, they will not necessarily be forthcoming. One carer speaks of the difficulty she had convincing the authorities that she really had got to the point of being unable to cope single-handed any longer.[19] Services to carers and/or their dependants are often discriminatory in application. A study of 172 carers[20] showed that 75 per cent of sons and 68 per cent of husbands received home help support as compared with only 4 per cent of mothers, 20 per cent of wives and 24 per cent of daughters. Where there is a carer, and she is a woman, there is no urgent need.

Government by Euphemism

'We now have government by euphemism: the priority groups are in fact the groups with the lowest priority; informal carers means unpaid women with few rights and little support; community care means "I think we can save a bit here".'[21] Community care as a policy for people with mental health problems seems to have different meanings for different people. Leaving the rest of us – past, present and potential recipients of services – aside, the government has a view of care by 'the community' where families look after their own and voluntary agencies become substantial service providers, while mental health professionals and pressure groups aim for care in 'the community' in dispersed local settings by redeployed (and, where necessary, retained) mental health workers. For others community care is an ideal yet to come, or an idea which lost its credibility a long time ago.

Whatever happens in practice, one thing is sure, that any failure in planning or provision will be paid for by the 'unpaid women with few rights and little support'. When the only alternative may be the streets or bed and breakfast hotels, or indeed the scarce council flat or hostel place, the pressure is on for people discharged from mental hospitals to live with their families regardless of whether that would usually be their choice (e.g. it may well not be where the 'dependant' is a parent or an adult daughter or son).

The closure of psychiatric hospitals, a process begun with the closure of Banstead in 1986, is going to increase greatly the number of people in need of supported housing (some 63,000 people are living in hospital), and increase both the necessity for good planning and the possibility of making drastic mistakes. Women are heavily enough implicated in the policy as it is; it is vital that failures in planning do not lead to outright exploitation.

Taking Action

There are a number of ways in which women's interests as carers are being served by various agencies and by themselves through mutual support.

First, any services which make it possible for people with mental health problems or other disabilities/frailties, to live as independently and autonomously as they are able, allow both family and the dependent person to choose whether or not to live together and so to opt in or out of the full 'caring relationship'. Projects such as those of the Stonham Housing Association in Southampton, show that people who are seriously disabled by their mental health problem can, with the right support, live independently of their families. Sheltered housing schemes with nursing services attached could care for quite dependent elderly people while maintaining maximum independence (independence of their families is what pensioners overwhelmingly want).[22] Services which provide refuge in times of crisis, meaningful daytime occupation and continuity of support, indirectly benefit carers as well as serving the direct recipient of the service.

There are also services and projects geared specifically to the informal carer, or the task of informal caring. Different kinds of support are possible, though all pale against the value of housing and income support directed to the dependent person. The carer can receive payment and that payment could be available to whoever was offering the service; the carer can be given backup in order to make their continued service possible; carers can meet together to give mutual support and air the anger and frustration which they may experience daily; carers can act together as a lobby to work for the kinds of services they can see are needed.

Paying Carers

A GP and social worker in a small Lancashire community are using attendance allowance to enable neighbours to visit regularly and play a substantial role in the care and supervision of three elderly women who are at different stages of dementia.[23] Two of the women live with members of their family; one lives alone. Under the scheme they are able to avoid admissions to hospital, which they would either resist or find distressing. More realistic payments to carers than the current state benefits would both value their service and recognize the loss in earnings which caring often entails. It would also provide a basis for enlisting the help of someone outside the family network, as in two of the instances in Lancashire. The carers' allowance – Invalid Care Allowance – is £23.75 a week (1988), plus £14.20 for an adult dependant or £8.05 for a child. Attendance Allowance, paid to the person in need of care, is £31.60 or £21.10 a week (day and night/day or night). Perhaps the main drawback from a woman's point of view is that the state is still relying on women's labour, this time low rather than unpaid. However it would materially improve the situation of the many women who are in fact undertaking caring work and allow the cared-for person more choice in and control over how they live.

Back-up for Carers

Carers support schemes are a very real lifeline for informal carers and, for their relatives, often mean the difference between admission to care and staying at home. They come in different shapes and sizes but the most praised seem to be so on the basis of their flexibility and capacity to provide the service that is actually wanted by the carer. Some schemes offer one kind of service in one kind of way (e.g. a volunteer sitting scheme) when that might not be the form of support many of the hard-pressed carers on their patch are wanting to take up. Some of the factors which influence that choice are: simple preference, infirmity of the carer, reluctance for a couple, for example, to regard themselves as carer and cared-for, reluctance to admit the need of help, acceptance by the dependent person, inhibition over asking for help, reluctance to leave the dependent person with a stranger, and reluctance to accept charity.[24]

The Crossroads Care Attendant Scheme provides home support including, where necessary, both domestic tasks and personal care of the dependent person. An evaluation of its services found that they are tailored to the expectations of carers and disabled person.[25]

A scheme in Sheffield aimed at supporting the relatives of people who are elderly and mentally infirm has concentrated on building up relationships between project workers and carers from which basis the actual requirements of carers can be established and met. As a result a variety of forms of support are offered rather than a single service. The scheme is based in a health centre (which means good access, and credibility), employs two local women as its part-time workers and has volunteers. It is another example of resources being used effectively to meet stated needs.[26]

The evaluation of Crossroads schemes noted what small amounts of support could enable carers to carry on. This kind of back-up could however result in women being able to cope, just, with high levels of stress, but not freed to pursue other avenues of their lives or compensated for the material loss their caring has given rise to. The obvious cost effectiveness of such schemes in keeping people out of residential care or hospital must not become a reason for keeping women at home and reinforcing the expectation that they will.

Carers Support Each Other

The value of support groups, and therapy for women in different situations, has been shown many times over. The White City project in West London for one has demonstrated the effectiveness of counselling and psychotherapy, by the decrease in the number of women visiting their doctors for tranquillizers and anti-depressants. Carer groups, typified by those developed by or affiliated to the Association of Carers, provide valuable space for carers' own needs to be acknowledged and met. A project in Islington North London has weekly meetings during which its members can share their frustration, exhaustion and depression, as well as express humour and their feelings of loyalty and reward. They have outings, which may be the only freedom they get, and they help each other through difficult times – whether enabling someone to decide to stop 'caring' without guilt, working through the grief, relief and guilt associated with the death of the dependent person, or encouraging someone to seek help with the task they have willingly taken on but cannot manage alone.[27]

Carers Fight Back

Carers as campaigners can bring the most authentic voice to planning bodies which effectively decide their fate. The same groups which provide mutual support may go on to lobby for change, and this is the case with the group in Islington. Indeed, nationally the Association of Carers is a pressure group and all the local groups connected with it strengthen its case, whether or not they have the time or energy to campaign themselves. However, local action is important, as that is where many decisions affecting the shape of services are made, and by winning representation on local forums and planning committees carers can ensure their needs get a hearing. It is by keeping up this pressure that women can avoid colluding in their own oppression as carers.

What do Women Want?

The first and most important answer to this question must be, 'to be asked'; the second, 'to be listened to'. Important as pressure groups and voluntary organizations are in focusing issues and extending the possibilities of what can be asked for, their opinions are not a substitute for those of the women at the receiving end of services, and planners and providers of services must learn to hand over some of their control of resources to the people who know best the effects of their deployment.

For the rest, here are some suggestions. Women who have dependent relatives want to be able to make choices that are tolerable; to choose out of love and loyalty to take on the bulk of the caring responsibility, without committing themselves to a life of intolerable strain; or to choose not to take on that responsibility without having to consign their relatives to unacceptable living conditions and thereby destroying the basis of love and loyalty that the relationship has. The poverty of life in hospitals, hostels and many residential homes forces many women to spend their lives caring for their relatives.

Women in their own right want: the choice of women-only space and services; the possibility of taking small children to whatever services they need to use; to be able to scream with rage and not be regarded as mad; to be able to give voice to despair, fear, exhaustion and extreme depression without losing their children; to be able to walk out of the GP's surgery clutching the number of a counsellor, a therapist, a support group, or a refuge instead of a tranquillizer prescription. Women want to have their confidence and self-esteem built up, not undermined, and to have the concrete actualities of their lives seen and acknowledged by anyone who is responsible for 'helping' them.

Notes

1. L. Eichenbaum and S. Orbach, *Understanding Women*, Penguin 1985, p. 9.
2. Women in MIND, *Finding our own Solutions*, MIND 1986, pp. 10, 13.
3. Ibid, p. 80.
4. From the song 'Ugly Little Dreams' by Everything But The Girl on *Love Not Money*, WEA Records 1985.
5. G. W. Brown and T. Harris, *Social Origins of Depression: A Study of Psychiatric Disorder in Women*, Tavistock 1978.
6. C. New and M. David, *For the Children's Sake*, Penguin 1985, p. 183.
7. I. K. Broverman and D. M. Broverman quoted in Irene Starr, 'The depressed sex?', *Social Work Today*, 26 August 1985, p. 16.
8. Women in MIND, *Finding our own Solutions*, p. 21.
9. S. Ahmed, 'Cultural Racism in Work with Women and Girls' in Transcultural Psychiatry Society, *Women: Cultural Perspectives: Conference Report*, TPS 1984, pp. 3–13.
10. Y. Alibhai, 'Culture Shocks', *New Society*, 28 November 1986, p. 11.
11. P. S. Penfold and G. A. Walker, *Women and the Psychiatric Paradox*, Open University Press 1984, pp. 83–4, 180.
12. Equal Opportunities Commission quoted in P. Beresford and S. Croft, *Whose Welfare?*, Lewis Cohen Urban Studies Centre 1986, p. 116.
13. J. Finch, 'Community care and the Invisible Welfare State', *Radical Community Medicine*, Summer 1986, p. 15.
14. Ibid., p. 17.
15. A. Briggs, *Who Cares? The Report of a Door-to-Door Survey into the Numbers and Needs of People Caring for Dependent Relatives*, Association of Carers 1983, p. 12.
16. Beresford and Croft, *Whose Welfare?*, p. 124.
17. M. Cooper, 'On the right road', *Community Care*, 14 August 1986, pp. 24–5.
18. Paul Reading, *Relatively Speaking*, Oxford MIND 1986, p. 20.

19. R. Cowling in A. Briggs and J. Oliver, *Caring: Experiences of Looking After Disabled Relatives*, Routledge and Kegan Paul 1985, p. 6.

20. Equal Opportunities Commission, *Caring for the Elderly and Handicapped: Community Care Policies and Women's Lives*, EOC 1982, p. 33.

21. C. Heginbotham, 'Life after Mental Illness? Opportunities in an Age of Unemployment' in *Life after Mental Illness? ... Major Papers from MIND's 1984 Annual Conference*, MIND 1985, p. 7.

22. Harris Research Centre Survey quoted in Beresford and Croft, *Whose Welfare?*, p. 138.

23. C. Grimshaw, 'Keeping Out of Hospital', *OPENMIND*, No. 8, April/May 1984, pp. 8–9.

24. J. Green, 'A break or a breakdown?', *Community Care*, 15 May 1986, pp. 22–4.

25. Cooper, 'On the right road', p. 25.

26. Green, 'A break or a breakdown?'.

27. Women in MIND, *Finding our own Solutions*, pp. 106–9.

5

Black People, 'Dangerousness' and Psychiatric Compulsion

ERROL FRANCIS

The aim of these extracts from interviews with lawyers working in the field of mental health is to widen the debate that has been taking place around black people and the psychiatric services. This debate began as far back as the late 1970s when Raymond Cochrane published his analysis of the 1971 census figures which indicated a large over-representation of black people as psychiatric patients, and a massive over-diagnosis of schizophrenia.[1] But it was not until 1981 that the debate started in earnest with the publication of Lipsedge and Littlewood's *Aliens and Alienists* which began to apply sketchy statistical and case-historical proof to what was by then a worsening picture.[2]

It was becoming increasingly clear that black people were being over-diagnosed as psychotically dangerous (rather than neurotic); were more likely to be admitted to hospital under compulsory procedures – especially by means of section 136 of the Mental Health Act which provides for police apprehension of people thought to be suffering from mental illness; and that black people, once in hospital, tended to be incarcerated in the locked and secure facilities. Furthermore it also began to be noticed that treatment of black patients was substantially inferior – psychotropic medication appeared to be given in larger doses, in the absence of less physically destructive treatments like psychotherapy – than that accorded to white patients.

What amounts to a major crisis in health care and social services provision to the black community has been given scant attention by policy-makers and academics. There is a dearth of substantive research which concentrates on the true extent of the crisis, let alone the reasons for the apparently massive psychiatrization of blacks and the mounting evidence of abusive treatment and punitive neglect. The revision of the 1959 Mental Health Act into the current 1983 legislation came too early on in the black community's awareness of the problem so that no meaningful demands were made for the legislation to be revised with black people in mind.

But perhaps this inaction is not surprising when one considers the limited conception that has been given to what constitutes 'the psychiatric system' anyway, and therefore the precise manner in which black people have been interacting with it. Indeed, the connection that black people have with psychiatry has tended to be viewed very narrowly as focusing on the hospital. This approach ignores some crucial links between the various institutions in this society. The psychiatric system, as Castels et al.[3] have pointed out, is a complex network of scientific expertise and professional practice which covers many areas of social life and permeates various institutions.

If one extends the conception of the psychiatric system to include schools, hospitals, social services, courts and prisons, then a very different map can be drawn of the relationship of black people to psychological knowledge and psychiatric practice. For a start, it brings into perspective the long-held concern of the black community that the quasi-eugenic practice of IQ testing is diagnosing more black schoolchildren as educationally subnormal (ESN). And this concern should be extended to include those black children who are deemed emotionally maladjusted or suffering from personality disorders. There seems therefore to be a legitimate case for investigating the involvement of black children with school psychology[4] (and parapsychology in remedial provisions for the disruptive and backward) as part and parcel of the problem of psychiatrization because it could well be that the school is the beginning of the psychiatric histories of many black people.

There is now also a pressing need to examine psychiatry's function within the criminal justice system. Little notice has been taken, either by commentators on mental health or by activists concerned with the criminalization process, of psychiatry as a sentencing option in the courts along with its traditional role of advising courts on criminal motivation. The result of this duality has been what appears in many cases to be a coalescence of criminalization and medicalization of black people – a coalescence which has gone largely unopposed.

The observations made in these interviews which follow are not backed up by statistical evidence; rather, they are based on trends that are only just beginning to be noticed about sentencing patterns and the involvement of psychiatry with black people passing through the courts. Nevertheless, ·the proof would seem axiomatic: if, as everyone knows, the criminal justice system draws in proportionally more blacks than any other group, then psychiatry must be coming into contact with black people with great frequency simply by virtue of the prominence of forensic psychiatry in the assessment and sentencing of criminality.[5]

Prison psychiatry also needs to be scrutinized. Alarm has been expressed about the use of tranquillizers for control reasons. A recent House of Commons Social Services Committee[6] which looked into the Prison Medical Service also voiced concern over the medical services to prisoners in general, and the psychiatric services in particular. They admitted that the latter were sometimes used on the instigation of the discipline staff controlling 'disruptive' prisoners.

There have been several well-publicized cases of black people being transferred from prison to special hospitals or given psychiatric treatment in gaol for what turned out to be punitive reasons.[7]

Finally the police are brought into play with their access to psychiatric compulsion via section 136 of the Mental Health Act. This empowers them to apprehend anyone in a public place who appears to be mentally ill, and to take them to a 'place of safety' (which can be a police station or a hospital) for psychiatric assessment. Because of widespread concern that section 136 is being over-used in metropolitan areas some research is being carried out now to measure the extent of the problem.

It has now been clearly established that the police are over-sectioning black people,[8] although the explanations that have been put forward tend to absolve the police of intentional criminalization/medicalization (i.e. of using section 136 as the mental health form of 'sus') and to put the abuses down to unconscious cultural bias. However, the wealth of evidence now showing the inappropriateness of police involvement in mental health matters has not led to a sustained campaign for the abolition of section 136. Clearly, then, there is need for more open discussion of the issues and for these discussions to be led by black people rather than by professional liberals.

In these interviews we discuss two aspects of the problem briefly outlined above: dangerousness and compulsion, because it is on this axis that much of psychiatric decision-making rests – the degree of risk posed by mentally ill people. Through analysing several cases that were notable at the time for the manner in which the assessment of dangerousness and the exercise of compulsion were intertwined, we try to raise questions about the cause of these abuses of black patients and whether they were accidental, 'cultural', or part of the structural and normal way that the system operates.

What is notable in the cases we discuss, is that the over-assessment of psychiatric dangerousness in black people is leading to the use of such excessive force that the psychiatric response itself becomes indistinguishable from forcibly imposed law and order. Through a desire not to forget (rather than through a desire for martyrdom) we recall the cases of Paul Worrell, Winston Rose, Colin Roach and others whose deaths and the destruction of whose lives are connected in some way or other with forms of psychiatric intervention that were either wholly unnecessary or were pitifully inadequate.[9]

Extracts from an interview with Gareth Pierce, Solicitor, on 9 June 1986:

G.P. : Both Winston Rose and Paul Worrell were people who were very impressive on a personal level and would be extremely valuable members of the community. They are both dead at the hands of the authorities in all sorts of ways and they were never accorded any degree of professionalism in terms of dealing with them. It was just the crudest possible approach to two people who were each going through a period of some sort of crisis.

Winston Rose

G.P.: Winston Rose was undergoing some sort of mental pressure at the time which was causing him, in his wife's view, to suffer from delusions. He believed that he was receiving some sort of sign that he was being observed or bugged. A lot of people during their lives undergo periods of crisis or trauma or have some sort of combination of circumstances that can cause a psychotic episode.

In his wife's view, Winston Rose needed more help than she could give him. She very properly went to see his doctor to ask for help. Now after that arose a situation in which all the authorities who dealt with him were in some way or other reprehensible. His general practitioner appears not to have given sufficient thought to the method by which he ought to have been detained in a mental hospital. The social services and the psychiatrists were also brought in and the police who were called in to actually effect his apprehension.

Now he was a gentle man who had never displayed violence towards his family or anybody else. He was, at the time that they were seeking to take him to a mental hospital, sitting in his shed at the bottom of his garden reading his Bible. He was jumped on by police who held him round the throat for a period of time until he died. They held him round the throat in an illegal neck hold and literally choked him to death. He was carried off through his neighbour's garden dead and put on the floor of the police van. They claim that they did not realize until the van was on its way that he was dead.

This was a man who wasn't a criminal, wasn't a danger to

anybody or to himself. You would have thought that anybody who had any sanity would have understood that this
sort of person was in a period of crisis and needed the utmost
sympathy, support and caring help towards treatment. Instead
of which he had police unleashed on him who said they had
no direction at all of what they were meant to be doing. One
of them said at the inquest, 'All I knew was that he was big
and coloured'. And it was that crude and racist approach on
behalf of everybody who dealt with him, that led to his
dying.

Why couldn't an ambulance have been called and his wife,
who deeply cared for him, be asked to sit in the ambulance
with him, together with trained, medical people? Why were
the police brought in with their known attitudes and why
then did they jump on him when he was no danger to anybody? It was a most disgraceful situation. The inquest jury
came up with a verdict of unlawful killing which means, and
this is the way that they were directed [by the coroner], that
the negligence of those concerned was so extreme that it
wasn't lack of care – it became unlawful killing.

But to the best of our knowledge nothing has ever happened to discipline any of those people who were involved in
his death. One would include here the doctors and the local
authority.

E.F.: When did this happen?

G.P.: 1981.

E.F.: How was this action authorized? How did the police come
to be in Winston Rose's garden?

G.P.: Under the Mental Health Act it is permitted for the police
to be brought in to assist in detaining somebody. But after
the experience of Winston Rose one really asks whether it is
appropriate for them to be brought in, when ambulance men
are obviously trained in more humane and safer methods of
restraint – if restraint is needed. But there is absolutely no
evidence that restraint was even needed. How did anyone
know that Winston wouldn't go? Nobody asked him . . .

As I understand it, Winston's case was meant to have led to

some changes or recommendations [in the 1983 Mental Health Act]. Certainly the coroner, at the end of the inquest, made a number of recommendations, to be followed in the future, about the ways in which people are dealt with. But one feels that if Winston Rose had been white he would have been dealt with in a different way. It was the attitudes of all the people involved ... The police officer was probably being very honest when he said, 'All I knew was that he was big and coloured', because that was all any of the authorities had thought it relevant to tell the police, as if that's somehow of any relevance at all.

E.F.: In what particular ways do you think that racism affected the way that the various agencies involved in this incident treated Winston Rose, especially the GP, social services and the police – the crucial people in actually effecting compulsory detention under the Mental Health Act?

G.P.: As I remember it, there was an assumption – it wasn't spelled out – that because this man was black, he had to have this huge barrage of police to detain him. It seemed implicit that he couldn't be regarded as gentle, although there was no evidence to show that he wasn't ... The only explanation that can somehow be erected – for what ended up as a mass police presence and somebody being killed – is that everybody had a completely wrong perception of, I wouldn't say the 'individual' because I don't think they saw him as an individual, but of the situation they were dealing with. That devastating comment by one of the officers, 'All I knew was that he was big and coloured', says a lot. Whoever relayed that information was relying, in my view, on a shorthand, racist code-message. There's no other explanation for it.

E.F.: 'All I knew was that he was big and coloured' contains no clear identification of this man as being distressed rather than criminal ...

G.P.: In that situation the information that could have been passed on is, 'He's a family man. He's in his own garden. He doesn't seem to be causing any trouble. His wife is in the house and a social worker is there. He's someone who has no previous psychiatric history. We think that the police probably aren't going to be needed but would you just be nearby but not show yourselves in case you frighten him.'

E.F.: The policeman's message is concerned with physical size and an associated threat ... ?

G.P.: That's explicit white racism isn't it? And certainly in the immediate reports that were put out afterwards, Winston was a foot taller – well that's because they'd killed him. That's absolutely classical white racism!

E.F.: In this situation that particular comment authorizes the use of force because it says there's a threat ...

G.P.: It's like an incitement ...

E.F.: ... to force?

G.P.: Yes. Provided you know that the recipient of that [message] is going to be prejudiced along those lines.

E.F.: So would you say that the major issue that is brought out by the death of Winston Rose is the amount of force that was used to deal with a situation which was not in itself threatening?

G.P.: It was completely inappropriate that he was not dealt with by the ambulance services with a familiar face in attendance ... Instead of that he was killed, handcuffed – his hands behind his back – and thrown face-down on the floor of the van. When it became apparent that he was dead, artificial respiration couldn't be properly applied because the officers in the van did not have the key to undo the handcuffs. It was a horrific series of negligent acts. And all you can assume from the whole catalogue was that not one person saw this man as an individual in desperate need of caring help.

Paul Worrell

G.P.: Paul Worrell was a boxer and I knew him before he died. Paul was a kind, gentle person and should never have been in a prison at all – that was quite outrageous. His parents thought he probably needed some help before his arrest because he was hearing voices and he had jumped out of a window. He then was arrested for having stabbed somebody. This was completely out-of-character. He had no previous convictions. He was remanded in custody at Brixton Prison and was given no help. The prison said he was not suffering from any mental illness. He was then seen by a psychiatrist for his defence, who, after talking to him and his family (which is something that the prison doctor never did) diagnosed him as suffering from schizophrenia. He should then have been transferred to a mental hospital where he could have been treated ... he would be here today.

Instead of that he was left locked up 24 hours a day in Brixton Prison in solitary confinement. He was even put on punishment at one stage. It was a lay member of the Board of Visitors – a black member – who decided that he was not well, when in fact the doctors at Brixton Prison were not even bothering to recognize his illness. Shortly before he was due to go to a mental hospital – while he was locked up and dosed on Largactil – he hanged himself. His family feels that we'll never know the full truth about what happened.

The coroner at the inquest told the jury that there was only one verdict that they could come to, and that was suicide. I objected. The evidence had been by no means clear, including utter negligence on the part of the prison. The jury came to an open verdict! So there's clear and worrying evidence that everything that happened to Paul Worrell – whether he took his own life or not – was someone else's failure. Once again this was an avoidable death.

E.F.: There was a similar case last year, at Strangeways Prison in Manchester, where a man who was ill and had been in prison on remand for quite a while, was found hanged in his cell.

G.P.: There are a troubling number of deaths in that category. There was another young man in Ashford Remand Centre called James Heather Hayes ... very similar. Often it is people at that age when life is extremely difficult – you're emerging from childhood and becoming an adult ... That's the time when many young people have nervous breakdowns or have acute forms of difficulty. They are regularly incarcerated in completely inappropriate conditions.

Here was this extremely impressive young man whom the prison clearly failed to recognize as such or as a human being. If they had, they would have seen all the warning signs; they would have seen that he was someone who might well take his own life. They failed to categorize him as a suicide risk even though the police had said that he had jumped out of a window before: even though he had cut his face with a razor while he was in Brixton; and even though he was deeply depressed, they had him locked in a cell for the whole time with bars at a height where it was most convenient for him to hang himself.

We asked psychiatrists before the inquest about treatment of someone who is schizophrenic. They said that treatment would probably be two-pronged. You might make use of a major tranquillizer which would calm down the aspect of delusions and allow you to treat the individual. The other more important prong, however, would consist of involving the person in therapy and relationships with other people because what had broken down was their ability to deal with people. You would rebuild that in the context of activity. When asked what was the worst possible situation the psychiatrists answered that it was 'to leave them on their own' ...

E.F.: The problem of psychiatry in prisons is contradictory, isn't it? On the one hand you have lots of cases of people who are ill, as in the case of Paul Worrell, and they cannot get help inside the prison. But on the other hand you have cases where prisoners are diagnosed as mentally ill and treated with tranquillizers for control reasons.

G.P.: The kind of psychiatric approaches in prison are inevitably crude because there aren't the trained people and there aren't the resources. But prison isn't appropriate for most people who are there ...

E.F.: I would now like to ask you about the assessment of 'dangerousness' and the involvement of psychiatry in the legal process.

G.P.: If someone is mentally ill at the time that they commit an offence and would not have offended had they not been mentally ill at the time, then the court ought to be interested in disposal and treatment rather than punishment. But as things stand at the moment, the courts' primary concern appears to be to lock up people whom they consider a danger to the community, particularly in the remand period.

I have been in front of courts applying for bail for someone to be treated and I've pointed out to the magistrate that the person is likely to commit suicide and have heard the magistrate say, 'That is not our concern'. Equally, we've been to prisons and said, 'We think if the defendant for whom we act remains in the situation they are in in prison, they're unlikely to survive to the trial'. And the prison authorities have said, 'That is not down to us'. In that triumvirate of power there seems to be an extraordinary ability to pass the buck in terms of acknowledging that this person ought to be a patient. The doctors, the courts, the prisons and, to an extent, the police all say, 'It's not our problem; all we can do is ensure that this person continues in custody in prison because the most important interest is that of the community at large.'

The paramount consideration is danger to others. If the greater danger is to himself or herself, that somehow manages to be downgraded because of two things. Firstly, the courts will not force the issue and demand that appropriate care be provided and secondly, the National Health Service simply will not build appropriate facilities. For the most part they don't exist. The catchment areas in London for example are so difficult for people to qualify for help that sometimes they can't get the right treatment because of where they live or where they were arrested. But that still begs the question whether the care and treatment where it exists is responsive to people's needs.

If you compound all that with the racism of society anyway and the inadequacies in relation to all mentally ill people, the overall picture for black people is very bad.

Extracts from an interview with Edward Fitzgerald, Barrister, on 3 July 1986:

E.F.: The predominant concern about mental illness in this country is whether the afflicted individuals are a threat to others rather than a threat to themselves. This is significant when one comes to talk about black people, because diagnosing a psychotic condition runs parallel with other characterizations of black people – as being aggressive, as being irrational, and so on ... Isn't there a lot that psychiatry is doing at the moment which makes it complicit with the criminalization of black people by the police?

Ed. F.: Well, the evidence shows that the over-representation of black people in mental hospitals is primarily in relation to compulsory detention, which is significant. Obviously compulsory detention is where the fear of 'threat to others' is going to play the biggest part. I can give you an example.

It's a case of a person I met in Broadmoor, who'd been in a local mental hospital – Claybury – where he had attacked a nurse. Now he was thought to be unmanageable in Claybury, and though he'd never been convicted of any criminal offence, he was sent to Broadmoor, where he was consistently diagnosed in a very negative way and finally spent ten years in the hospital without having exhibited any florid symptoms of mental illness for some time, and without having been particularly dangerous or aggressive on the ward. The element of fear as to what this person might do in the future seemed to be playing a major part.

An interesting thing was that the psychiatrist – actually an independent psychiatrist – went down to see this West Indian patient and said to him 'What are you going to do when you leave hospital?' He answered, 'Well the first thing I'm going to do is get myself a drink and find myself a woman.' Now that relatively innocent comment might well reflect a frank admisson of what's going on in most people's minds when they've been detained for ten years. But this was put forward as 'convincing evidence' that this person was a potential rapist – although there was no evidence of sexual assaults in the past. And that, I think, is an example of how racist factors are subconsciously playing on the mind. I don't believe that if it had been a white person who made that remark, in a white way ... that it would have been interpreted in that way.

E.F.: When we come to consider section 136 of the Mental Health Act there has been a lot of concern from the black community that in this section two things are coinciding: the fear of black crime in conjunction with the police being asked to make what is in effect a psychiatric judgement as to whether someone is mentally ill or not. Is this not a case of criminalizing and medicalizing?

Ed. F.: Well, again there's overwhelming evidence that black people are massively over-represented in section 136s, and one can't avoid conjecturing that it's something to do with police perceptions of black people. Certainly, on the criminalizing front, the perception of a black person who is acting 'bizarrely' as dangerous – rather than as someone who needs to be talked to and helped to seek out voluntary care – must play a large part. The medicalizing side of it may of course be because you've got amateurs trying to diagnose and I think it is reasonable to say that the symptoms that are picked up by the policeman may simply be the person behaving eccentrically ...

As to whether the policeman is as prepared, as in the case of a white person, to discuss voluntary treatment or to try to find some alternative way of sorting out the problem ... I think probably the fears of the police tend to make them jump to a section 136 sooner when the person is black. That may be a somewhat generous interpretation of what goes on in the police force, but they can't have any deliberate motive for wanting to put a section 136 on people. I think section 136 over-representation requires a look at the subconscious rather than the deliberate misinterpretations of the police force. But certainly the section 136 has been described as the mental health substitute for 'sus' ...

E.F.: What seems to be apparent in the operation of section 136 is two different forces: there is the legal and the psychiatric element and these seem to coincide with the definition of mental illness as being something which causes social disruption. A lot of people who are critical of psychiatry describe it as a form of social control in the same way that we would describe policing, even for positive reasons, as control. Do you not think that, in the case of section 136 psychiatry as a medical discipline and psychiatry as an apparent instrument of law and order have become unhelpfully confused?

Ed. F.: Well, I suppose the question is, if you abolished section 136 would the problem go away?

E.F.: It may be possible to separate psychiatry from this law and order element ...

Ed. F.: Giving the police the power to say that someone is mentally disordered, in their view, reflects on police attitudes rather than on psychiatry. After all, at that stage there is no psychiatrist involved.

I probably differ from many people discussing this issue in that, from a radical perspective, I actually do believe that there is an objective bedrock to Western psychiatry which one mustn't doubt. Once you start doubting that, then everything becomes purely relative ... It's dangerous to say that psychiatry is in itself an instrument of social control; it's psychiatry as used when you start sectioning people! Once you've got the compulsory sections of the Mental Health Act, obviously it becomes like imprisonment and a means of social control and that's where the dangers come in. Perhaps section 136 should be abolished altogether, because it is giving people who've got no knowledge of mental disorder a pretext for interfering. So that would be my objection to section 136.

E.F.: I was not trying to deny that there is schizophrenia, or that there is such a thing as mental illness. I was not taking an anti-psychiatry position, i.e. that mental illness does not exist except in the minds of those who diagnose it. What I was suggesting was that psychiatry, certainly of the kind that we have in the West, has chosen to align itself in a certain way with law enforcement ideas, or ideas which come very close to that, at the expense of exploring ways of genuinely helping people through these mental conditions. Is what black people are having to contend with a mere error in the system, or a hiccup in judgement – unconscious, as you say – or is it the result of something much deeper, going to the nature of psychiatry and its alignment with controlling institutions in the society, like the criminal justice system, for example?

Ed. F.: In making out a case for itself, psychiatry at some stage in history has tried to present itself as useful to the powers that be, and one sees this particularly in areas like psychopathy and mental impairment. Social judgements came out in the notion that medicine had something to offer in the sphere of mental handicap, for example. Now the attitude that the mentally impaired must be locked up and stopped from breeding, lends itself to all sorts of racist abuses. Again in the case of psychopathy, once you start claiming as a doctor that you have got some cure for 'personality problems' which result in 'irresponsible conduct' you will inevitably be enlisted or volunteer for a social control role. I think that the pseudo-medical areas of mental impairment and psychopathy are those where psychiatry perhaps is departing from its medical origins and becoming a pure instrument of social control.

In the sphere of psychosis, it is probably a problem that people that come into reactive psychotic conditions are more likely to be seen as suffering from an endogenous condition – and I suppose that does fit in with basic racist notions that there's something in the black man, inside, which is causing his illness, rather than that an exploration of the cultural history of that particular person is needed to see how the illness came about and to find out that it may just have been a reaction to intolerable circumstances.

In the prison context one sees time and time again, that what's happened is that a black person has been put in intolerable conditions, probably in solitary confinement, getting themselves into confrontations with the prison warders and with other prisoners and that this has in fact led to a temporary breakdown. Now this breakdown is sometimes understood by sympathetic psychiatrists as being merely a temporary reaction to intolerable stress; but at other times the breakdown is misinterpreted as evidence that the person has been schizophrenic all along and therefore needs long-term hospitalization in a special hospital.

There was a case I met in Broadmoor Hospital where the psychiatrist was sympathetic. The black person's notion that he had been persecuted and attacked by the police without reason was being put forward as evidence of a delusional, schizophrenic, persecution complex. The psychiatrist – who finally ended up treating him – to his credit said that having regard to what goes on in society, he had no doubt that many of these things which had been put forward as paranoid symptoms were reactions to what he'd actually experienced.

So I think that there certainly is that danger that psychiatry will be enlisted to label someone as schizophrenic when the symptoms are only short-term reactions to really appalling pressures and whose so-called paranoid symptoms may in fact be quite justifiable reactions to what's going on in their life.

And to give another example. There was a case, again from my experience at Broadmoor, where the Responsible Medical Officer had said that the West Indian person in question had no family interested in him, no contact with the outside world, and that he was an isolated individual without any support likely to come to him when he was released. At the tribunal no less than eight members of his family turned up – all of whom confirmed that they'd been in regular contact with him, and all of whom, quite surprisingly for any patient in Broadmoor, came up with different schemes for rehabilitation – realistic ones which they'd obviously thought out and planned. It was not only not true that he didn't have any outside support: he had the most impressive array of supportive relations, who visited him and were concerned about him. That was a classic example of a doctor just not having explored the social context. If he had, it may well be that those relatives who finally turned up at the tribunal and gave a great deal of background information would have helped him to clarify the extent to which the illness was reactive or not, and also to what extent the prognosis of dangerousness was reliable.

Notes

1. R. Cochrane, 'Mental Illness in Immigrants to England and Wales. An Analysis of Mental Hospital Admissions 1971', *International Journal of Social Psychiatry*, 1977, Vol. 12, pp. 25–35.
2. R. Littlewood and M. Lipsedge, *Aliens and Alienists: Ethnic Minorities and Psychiatry*, Penguin 1981.
3. R. Castels, F. Castels and A. Lovell, *The Psychiatric Society*, Columbia University Press (USA) 1982.
4. *Ethnic Census of School Support Centres and Educational Guidance Centres*, Inner London Education Authority Research and Statistics Branch, RS 784/81. *Educational Opportunities for All?* ILEA Research Studies 1985.
5. *Submissions to the House of Commons Social Services Committee on the Prison Medical Service*, National Association for the Care and Resettlement of Offenders 1985.
6. House of Commons Social Services Committee, *Report No. III on the Prison Medical Service*, House of Commons, Session 1985/86, No. 72.
7. E. Francis, 'How Did Michael Dean Martin Die?', *OPENMIND*, No. 13, February/March 1985. Also, the Adjournment Debate called by the Labour MP Gerald Bermingham to ask questions raised by the suspicious death of Michael Martin at Broadmoor special hospital in June 1984, in Hansard, 21 March 1986.
8. A. Rogers and A. Faulkner, *A Place of Safety*, MIND 1987.
9. For a fuller discussion of the issues raised in this chapter see E. Francis, 'Psychiatric Racism and Social Police' to be published by Hutchinson in a forthcoming volume entitled *Inside Babylon*.

Part III
Some Home Truths

6
Housing for All

CHRIS HOLMES

Housing provision in Britain is organized primarily to meet the
requirements of two-parent white families, with secure well-paid
jobs. The great majority of such households are owner occupiers.
The ideology of owner occupation promotes the image of self-
reliant individuals, securing a home of their own without
dependence on the state. The reality is that most owners benefit
from extraordinarily generous tax privileges and other benefits.
The most important is tax relief on mortgage interest payments,
which now costs more than £4,500 million annually – and with
the greatest benefits going to those with the highest incomes
and large mortgages. Other benefits include big discounts for
former council tenants exercising the 'right to buy'; exemption
from capital gains taxation; and access to huge loans from
building societies and banks at relatively cheap interest rates –
without the rigid controls on levels of borrowing which so
constrain public authorities, and often with opportunities for
diverting loans into other forms of consumer spending.

These benefits, however, are available only to people with
stable incomes of an adequate level. The low-paid, the unemployed, sick and disabled people have little chance of becoming
home owners. Single people find it more difficult because of
being reliant on only one income. And on the margins of owner
occupation are growing numbers of relatively low-income
households – including many from ethnic minorities – who have
bought their homes through lack of any alternative, and are
now experiencing great difficulty in coping with the repayments
or paying for repairs.

At the turn of the century the overwhelming majority of
households in Britain rented from private landlords. This

proportion has fallen remorselessly over the past 70 years – from 90 per cent of all households in 1914, to 60 per cent in 1945 and now to only 12 per cent (and much less still if housing association tenancies and tied accommodation are excluded).

In itself this decline is no cause for mourning. The private rented sector has always contained the greatest concentration of unfit, ill-equipped and badly maintained properties. Private tenants are most likely to be living in overcrowded and multi-occupied accommodation, to experience harassment and illegal eviction and to lack security of tenure. The erosion of Rent Act protection, through legal changes and landlords exploiting loopholes in the law, means that a large number of new lettings are insecure.

The problem arises because no satisfactory alternative exists for many of those households who would previously have looked to the privately rented sector – especially young people leaving home, people moving into a new area, those leaving hospital or prison, and those losing their previous accommodation as the result of the break-up of a relationship.

Since the 1920s public rented housing has ensured decent homes for large numbers of working-class households. More than five million tenants – almost three in ten of all households – rent from local authorities or New Towns. For many of those who could not afford to buy, council housing has represented the only hope of a satisfactory, self-contained home at a cost they could afford. At its best, it has provided attractive homes, in settled communities, at reasonable rents – and transformed the lives of people desperate to escape from damp, overcrowded slum housing or unable to get anywhere to live at all.

These achievements, however, have been marred by serious flaws. First, the management of local authority housing has developed in the ideological tradition of Victorian paternalism within the framework of centralized municipal bureaucracy. It has been a producer-dominated tenure, rather than a service shaped by the preferences and aspirations of the users. Secondly, it has been deeply conditioned by the dictates of scarcity. Since demand has always exceeded supply, bureaucratic rules were necessary to determine priorities over who gets housed. The pressures to build as many homes as cheaply and quickly as possible has resulted in mass housing 'solutions' of system-built estates.

And when these external constraints reinforced the value judgements of the professionals, the practice became still more deeply embedded with authoritarian and elitist attitudes. Architects and planners could impose their choices on the sort of homes that were built without any consultation with the people who would live in them. Housing managers could treat 'their' tenants as recipients of welfare hand-outs.

This combination of scarcity and authoritarianism has powerfully influenced the allocation of council housing. Most authorities have developed allocation procedures which have given priority to the needs of families with children, to elderly people and to those with long local residence – reflecting deeply-held assumptions about who is 'deserving'. Little importance has been given to the needs of groups such as single people of working age. There is also systematically documented evidence of discrimination against black people in the allocation of public housing. And hostility is shown to groups seen as 'deviant' – such as lesbians and gay men.

In some circumstances local authorities have a legal duty to provide accommodation: for people displaced by clearance or redevelopment and for those defined as being homeless as a result of emergency or in 'priority need' as defined under Part III of the 1985 Housing Act (formerly the 1977 Homeless Persons Act). This includes families with dependent children, pregnant women and other homeless people considered 'vulnerable' – for example, because of old age, mental or physical illness or handicap. The great majority of single people and childless couples are excluded.

The treatment of homeless people is still characterized more by the ethos and values of the Poor Law than the entitlement to social rights of a civilized democracy. The legislation effectively distinguishes the 'deserving' from the 'undeserving'. There are no controls over the standard of accommodation that is offered.

Special powers on so-called 'intentional homelessness' reflect punitive attitudes to those who can be held to have been responsible in some way for their homelessness. And there are no effective rights of enforcement for homeless applicants.

These flaws in the legislation are shaped by, and also reinforce, the damaging myths and stereotypes about homeless people, and the perceptions of the apparently competing claims of applicants who present themselves to local authorities as homeless. The assumption is that having to house homeless people is a regrettable necessity to comply with the council's statutory obligations (although teachers would not think of complaining that they have a class full of children with a legal right to be at school).

The typical image of homeless applicants is almost always negative: 'queue jumpers', 'newcomers', 'immigrants', 'feckless'. In contrast the claims of those on the council's waiting list are described in the language of law abiding, deserving legitimacy: 'local residents', in 'housing need' patiently 'waiting their turn'. In reality these distinctions are nonsense. The people on housing waiting lists and those who present themselves as homeless are more and more frequently the same people. Growing proportions of those on waiting lists are people forced to live temporarily with friends or relatives because they cannot obtain a place of their own.

Indeed the whole concept of a 'waiting list' is itself becoming an anachronism. It implies that there is somewhere to wait. Historically, it has been the privately rented sector which has provided this waiting room – even though it was often run-down, overcrowded and lacking amenities. There is now a massive hole in housing policy and provision – particularly for all those who cannot afford (and may not wish) to buy, and need somewhere to live urgently.

It has been especially in the network of hostels and bed and breakfast lodging houses that a grotesque parody of the home ownership market has been found. Until 1985 unemployed people claiming supplementary benefit had a right to the cost of board and lodging – in its own way, it had been available on demand. Yet since there was no rent control, no security of tenure and no control over standards, the owners of these commercial establishments were able to make vast profits at public expense by letting out squalid, overcrowded and often unsafe accommodation to homeless people. The irony is that it would be not only far better, but actually cheaper, to allow the local council to provide proper self-contained flats than to pay the cost of board and lodging to commercial landlords. The government's response, however, has not been to encourage the provision of permanent homes, but to take away even the fragile rights which existed – by the board and lodging regulations which impose new ceilings on the maximum benefit payable and limit the length of time most young people under 25 can claim benefit in any one area.

The inequalities in the housing market are deeply rooted in the structures of housing tenure, finance and legislation and in conventional attitudes to the provision of housing. Yet they have been made sharply worse since 1979 by the Conservative government. Whilst the cost of mortgage tax relief has more than trebled – from £1,500 million to over £4,500 million a year – subsidies to local authority housing have been halved – from £1,500 million to less than £800 million a year. The 'right to buy' has resulted in the loss of three quarters of a million council homes – mainly the more attractive ones with gardens (and practically none in the less desirable high-density flatted estates).

Public spending on housing has been cut more severely than any other area of social spending – from £6.7 billion in 1979/ 80 to £2.7 billion estimated in 1986/7. And the worst casualty has been the number of new homes built for rent, which has fallen from an average of 150,000 new dwellings being built by council and housing associations in the mid-1970s, to just over 100,000 in 1980 and only 40,000 in 1985.

Despite these massive cut-backs in the scale of public provision, there have been some areas of expansion. One example is the increase in the numbers of beds in small hostels and supportive shared housing projects provided by housing associations and voluntary agencies – a total of over 13,000 bed-spaces approved by the Housing Corporation since 1980. These developments have provided more satisfactory alternatives to some of the archaic institutional hostels and night shelters, and a growth in the availability of supported housing. Yet they too have been stigmatized by the structure of provision and the labelling of this type of accommodation. The nature of the funding has forced agencies to provide shared accommodation in specially designed schemes, when what many residents would prefer is some form of support in their own self-contained flat. Access to the projects requires residents to be defined as 'mentally ill', 'ex-hostel resident', 'young homeless' – often the very labels from which they want to escape. The terms 'special project' or 'special needs' themselves imply the need for different kinds of housing for a particularly vulnerable group, rather than one type of housing within a comprehensive range of accommodation of equal status.

What is needed is a radically different approach, based on the assumption that housing is a right for every member of the community. That right should not depend on how much money people have, or whether they have children, or whether a landlord considers them deserving.

That must mean a commitment to combat discrimination of every kind. In British society, it is black people and women of any colour who are most likely to be homeless and put in bed and breakfast. It is young people who are denied access to waiting lists, have to live on lower levels of benefit, and are forced to move from one area to another. It is refugees, ex-offenders, people with mental health problems, disabled people, lesbians and gay men, who experience discrimination in their access to housing. Statutory rights are essential to ensure fair access, to stop arbitrary evictions and to enforce decent conditions.

A central demand, therefore, must be for a Housing Rights Act, which seeks to secure the legal right to a safe and satisfactory home for every member of the community. This must include:

- a duty on local authorities to secure a home for all those in severe housing need, including people with nowhere to live or threatened with homelessness, those in overcrowded or unfit accommodation and those in severe medical need;

- the right to be considered for local authority housing, regardless of age, length of residence, religion or any other arbitrary reason;
- a duty on local councils to inspect regularly and to enforce minimum conditions of repairs, safety, amenities, overcrowding and management in all multi-occupied dwellings;
- a right to security for all tenants of non-resident landlords, closing the loopholes in the Rent Acts, and strong sanctions against harassment and unlawful eviction;
- protection for those who are victims of racial or sexual harassment, including effective action against the perpetrators;
- the right for tenants to have a greater say in how their homes are planned and run, with proper funding for tenants associations, provided they are representative.

To meet those rights, of course, local authorities will need resources. The new rights can only be implemented if authorities are freed from the present crippling constraints, and able to develop a comprehensive housing strategy for meeting the full range of needs in their area – including those forms of housing stress and hidden homelessness which are so often ignored.

It is unjust that people who buy their homes are able to borrow, in total, huge sums of money – over £20 billion last year – from banks and building societies without any hint of controls on the total level of lending, whilst local authorities, housing associations and housing co-ops are subject to the most rigid controls on capital spending. Yet the cost in lost tax revenue through relief on mortgage interest payments is far greater than the subsidies to social rented housing.

The principles for a socially just housing policy are clear: there should be no more controls on the freedom of social housing agencies to provide homes for rent than there are on private individuals or companies building or acquiring homes for owner occupation. To achieve this, the present artificial capital controls should be abolished – including the limits on the use of receipts from the sale of council homes, the rigid annual Housing Investment Programme allocations, and the project controls on new schemes.

The present system of housing subsidies should be reformed, in order to create fairness between owners and tenants, and to ensure that subsidies go to the areas with the most severe problems and the people with the greatest need. This will mean redistributing mortgage tax relief, improving the housing benefit system and channelling housing investment subsidies to the housing stress areas. In the present climate those demands may seem idealistic – yet they are simple fairness and commonsense. It is only the shibboleths of the Treasury and archaic financial dogma which justify such illogical inequalities on different forms of housing provision.

A campaign to secure housing as a right for all, faces enormous obstacles: the power of entrenched privilege and the pursuit of profit, deeply ingrained prejudices over how people should live and who is deserving, and the lack of enforceable legal rights to safe, secure and satisfactory housing. It will be changed only through determined struggle, drawing together the different groups who experience oppression, and demanding the fundamental changes in laws, policies and attitudes that are needed.

7

Home after Hospital

RON THOMSON

Community care is not working, it is claimed,[1] and we should therefore call a halt to the projected closure of the old Victorian lunatic asylums. The fear is that running down these institutions will only increase the already large numbers of homeless people with mental health problems.

What informs these pessimistic statements is the fact that successive governments – Tory and Labour alike – have done nothing to help the community care for those vulnerable people who are always potentially homeless. Yet as far back as 1929 Dr E. O. Lewis, in a study of residents of casual wards – the name given to large reception centres prior to the 1948 National Assistance Act – found that 40 per cent had some form of 'mental disorder'.[2]

Research carried out in Camberwell Reception Centre (South London) during the mid-1960s concluded that it was then acting as a cheap low-care form of psychiatric hospital.[3] And now that the first series of hospitals are closing down, there is increasing evidence of people being discharged to hostels for single homeless people or to nowhere.

One Salvation Army officer told me how a couple of days ago he had looked out of his office window and seen an ambulance pull up. The driver got out, walked to the back doors of his ambulance, opened up and pointed to the hostel entrance. Two men then started walking towards the hostel. On questioning them, the officer discovered that both had just been discharged from Tooting Bec, a large psychiatric hospital in South London. Hospital staff had not been in touch with the hostel to check if they were prepared to accept the men as residents, or to see if the care was appropriate, or even if the hostel had two beds

89

available. This hostel employs no trained social workers or psychiatric nurses, and had been unsuccessful in its attempts to establish a regular liaison with either the social services department or the community psychiatric nursing service. So much for the planned discharge programme called for in the Short Report on Community Care.[4]

A survey later carried out in that same hostel, by a medical research team based at London's Guy's Hospital, found that up to 75 per cent of the residents had either existing or recent past histories of psychiatric hospital admissions. They wrote, 'This is an important new finding, which was not previously recognized.'[5] This was not news to those of us who have regular contact with the residents of those hostels, or who care to read previous studies on the subject! Why were the experts so surprised this late in the hospital closure programme?

Stories such as the one by the Salvation Army officer are quite common. In their report *Discharged into the Community*, Charlie Legg and Ada Kay recount the incident of a hospital patient being told that he would have to move out that day as the bed was needed that night.[6]

If the US experience is anything to go by, mentally vulnerable people in this country might be in for a rough ride. There, the hospital closures programme started in earnest in the 1960s and it resulted in very large numbers of people with mental health problems becoming homeless. In New York alone it was estimated that 36,000 homeless people were out on the streets, living in nightshelters, subways and abandoned buildings, with over 50 per cent of them suffering from a 'significant mental disability'.[7] Yet as one of the most thorough research reports indicated, 'It was not the concept of deinstitutionalization, but its implementation that was flawed.'[8]

Interestingly, Larry Gostin, Professor of Health Law at Harvard University, pointed out that it was Ronald Reagan, when he was Governor of California, who was the first to establish the policy of deinstitutionalization as a cost-saving measure . . .[9]

Individual Choices for Individual Needs

At the same time as hospitals are being run down, the DHSS
reception centres and a number of large hostels are closing.
Many of these large institutions have become home to people.
For example, in yet another Salvation Army hostel the officer
produced records which showed that 14 women had been in the
hostel for over 20 years (one for 32 years) and 40 for over ten
years. People who have lived in one place for so long need to be
offered an incentive of a better way of life to induce them to
move elsewhere. Yet what is happening? Often they are not
even consulted. The closure of Banstead hospital in Epsom,
Surrey resulted in most of the patients being transferred to
another hospital a few miles down the road.[10]

A similar picture is painted by Alison Wertheimer who found
that 74 per cent of the patients of mental handicap hospitals
which closed between 1979 and 1985 were moved to other
institutions.[11]

There is a further anomaly; the Poor Law of 1601 stipulated
that people had to return to their parish of origin for relief. This
is still in operation to a certain extent and again limits the individual's choices. We still see people leaving hospital and having
to return to the town or borough where they were living 20
years earlier because that is where they belong! That particular
local authority still has responsibility for them. This could mean
the break-up of friendships and relationships with local shopkeepers, church groups, pub and bingo clientele, forged while
people were living in the hospital.

When efforts are made to develop new types of accommodation, it is common for schemes to be planned without reference
to what would really suit the people who will live in them or what
would truly improve the quality of their lives. Instead, the money
available is frequently the only criterion. For example, a night
shelter for homeless people is worth establishing but if it is in
the crypt of a church – a place designed and built for storage of
dead bodies – the message is neither positive nor life-enhancing.

Many vulnerable people, particularly mentally ill or handi-capped people, are grouped together in settings which make it difficult to have personal space and privacy; they might have to share rooms even if they do not wish to; space for personal be-longings might be very limited; and they certainly cannot decorate the place to their taste. What they eat, when they eat and where, is decided by staff. Residents are not allowed in the kitchen as this would not be safe! Rules have to be adhered to and no exceptions can be made. Some hostels allow access to bedrooms only at limited times – a gate at the foot of the stairs is unlocked by a member of staff at set times and those may not coincide with the time you get in from work, dirty or sweaty. If you miss the 8.00pm opening you are trapped upstairs or downstairs till the 8.30pm opening. I know, because I lived in one for a year.[12]

Our home is where we are meant to feel most at ease, to be seen and respected for what we are, and to be ourselves. How can a person regain or keep a feeling of self-worth if he or she is treated without the respect due to an individual?

Types of Accommodation

A research study report produced in 1983 for the Department of the Environment[13] highlights the need for a wide range of housing provision including: (1) fully staffed hostels for re-habilitation; (2) low-staffed hostels for resettlement; (3) staffed and un-staffed group homes; (4) bedsitters or flats with com-munal facilities; (5) clustered self-contained units for one or two people; (6) ordinary flats.

There are, I would suggest, a number of alternatives within each of the above categories and as many ways of linking the support needs of the person to that of the housing design. How-ever there are problems attached to introducing any form of specialized accommodation and the more specialized the bigger the problems. Here are just some:

● a more sophisticated selection technique will have to be devised to meet narrowed criteria of eligibility;

- more gaps will be left for people to fall through;
- a person whose circumstances change for better or worse is more likely to find himself or herself under pressure to move elsewhere.[14]

This last point is worth expanding. Research has shown that moving house is ranked very high in the league table of stressful life events. Yet people seen as vulnerable are subject to a conveyor belt of moves, from the initial hospital ward, to the rehabilitation ward, to a hostel, to a group home, to a supported flat or bed-sitter, to an ordinary house or flat.

Each move along this conveyor belt seems almost deliberately designed to weed out the weak from the strong; many break down before the end of the journey. As the person moves from one environment to another, support is withdrawn and replaced by different, less intense types of assistance.

But why subject someone to a conveyor belt when, with just a bit more effort, he or she could be helped to build a support network around their 'ordinary' home? Systems such as Core and Cluster, DISH, Floating Support and others are now being designed to counteract this unsuitable move-on system.

The next section takes a more detailed look at some existing provision and projects.

Therapeutic Communities

My own experience of living and working in a therapeutic community of 20 residents and five staff serves only to illustrate how not to promote independence and self-determination. The theory was that all decisions on issues that affected the running of the house would be made by residents. In reality the decisions were made in the staff team meeting, whilst at the same time plans were worked out as to how we would ensure the same decisions would be reached in the full community meeting of residents and staff. The minor issues, however, were left solely to residents with some guidance from staff.

At the same time, I was supervisor/manager of a block of ten move-on flats owned by a local housing association. The tenants often saw it as an annexe to the hostel, as the same therapeutic philosophy was meant to be practised – matters which affected the running of the house were to be discussed in the weekly (compulsory) community meeting.

The introduction of two 'outsiders' – people who had not been through the main hostel – helped to break the annexe feeling. A slow, subtle change from a weekly two-hour therapy meeting for residents in the communal room, to a half-hour tenants' meeting followed by a socialization evening in the local pub introduced a different atmosphere. People started to feel more valued and, I believe, their self-image started to change. They were becoming friends rather than clients, tenants rather than residents. And my role was becoming that of facilitator rather than of a therapist.

The differences between the therapeutic community and the annexe set me thinking. And I became convinced that the inward-looking idea of 'building a community in a house' is definitely not the same as 'building a home in the community'.

Teaching someone to live with 25 others and to shop and cook for them, does not equip a person afterwards to live alone in a self-contained flat ...

Group Homes

The name 'group home' has a very wide usage, covering many different types of projects. Consequently when they are discussed in case conferences, usually as a next step after hospital for a patient who is about to leave, everyone has a different image.

The model of the 1960s was of a number of people from the same hospital ward going to live in the same house, all sharing the budget, cooking, cleaning, etc., although on occasion one of the residents would be expected to act as unofficial housekeeper for the others. This model (which I refer to as an Artificial Family Unit or AFU) proved to be successful for moving large numbers of long-stay institutionalized patients into the community. The key was that people had known each other for years on the ward.

The success of the AFU model, however, has led to the idea of bringing together people from different wards or from the wider community. These people may not even know each other, yet they are expected to share in the same way as in the AFU. When this fails it is often the resident who is blamed – he or she is a troublemaker, or a difficult person – rather than the set-up itself.

In circumstances such as these, when people do not know each other well, a shared house rather than a group home, might be a better solution. Each person can then live independently, sharing some facilities such as a kitchen and lounge. As the DoE report, referred to above, concludes, group homes 'are a convenient and low-cost form of provision for agencies to make, but it is not necessarily what the majority of mentally ill or mentally handicapped people need or want.'[15]

Core and Cluster

Core and Cluster schemes are designed to break away from the conveyor-belt systems as described earlier. If the resident's needs for support change, he or she stays while the staff move, either increasing or decreasing the support, or changing the type of assistance, e.g. a counsellor instead of an occupational therapist.

The core is an administrative base for the service. The cluster provides a range of accommodation spread throughout a neighbourhood (not a campus) using ordinary houses in a residential area and thus blending into the community without drawing attention to itself. Since the introduction of the concept in the ENCOR project in Nebraska, US, some years ago, it has been fine-tuned by other practitioners.

Its widely publicized success has however led to a number of service planners designing what they term as 'core and cluster', but which in effect reflects a somewhat distorted understanding of the initial concept. And the reaction to this threw up alternatives such as DISH. Each letter clearly spells out the aims of the concept. Dispersed: over a fairly large community. Intensively Supported: with the capacity to provide full seven-day 24-hour cover if necessary. Housing: the emphasis is on normal housing not hostels. The first of these which is being developed for elderly people with mental health problems, is a joint project between North West MIND, South Sefton Health Authority and Sefton Social Services.

However, a scheme set up in the style of a 'core and cluster' or DISH can still be a mini-institution unless efforts are made fully to integrate people into the natural community.

Training House

Much of the criticism levelled at the use of 'ordinary housing' for people with mental health problems is that they are still isolated in the community. They feel dumped into self-contained flats without friends, caring relatives or adequate skills for dealing with the day-to-day business of shopping, cooking, going to the launderette, budgeting, dealing with authorities.

One solution adopted by a local voluntary group in which I was involved was to set up a skills training house. The aim was to look at the full range of needs of residents and plan an individual development programme for each person to help them either to learn new skills or to revive and practise old ones which had not been needed in the institutions where they previously lived.

Looking back on this project the original planners realized that it was flawed to a certain extent as people had to move on into their new flat or bedsitter, and start all over again.

A second project which was set up at about the same time with a local housing association, was better tailored to people's needs. Our group signed a three-year management agreement on a house split into three self-contained flats. The aim was to provide and encourage skills training as the new residents were settling into their accommodation. At the end of the three years the residents would then be expected to have learned enough and not to need the intensive housing management skills which our group had been providing. The house would then formally be handed back to the housing association in exchange for another to keep the process going and help to ensure further integration into the natural community.

By using a number of ordinary people in this retraining process and normal community resources such as libraries, further education colleges, sports centres, the intention is to build up support networks of friends and neighbours around the person. The same sort of support that ordinary people have and use even if this is not formally recognized. The support networks are of course, additional to the services provided by statutory agencies, not in place of them.

The philosophy behind the projects that I would qualify as 'good practice', and which informs my criticism of others, is easy to summarize. It is that people no matter what their problem deserve to be treated as responsible individuals who have varying needs, interests and wishes; that there is no such thing as a group solution – all of us need choices; and finally that respect is an essential ingredient of 'good practice'.

Notes

1. Diana Brahams and Dr Malcolm Weller, 'Crime and Homelessness among the Mentally Ill', *New Law Journal*, 28 June and 26 July 1985. Monica Brimacombe, 'Dumping the Mentally Ill', *Roof Magazine*, November/December 1986.
2. *Relief of the Casual Poor*, HMSO 1930, Cmd No. 3640 xviii 121.
3. Griffith Edwards et al., 'Census of a Reception Centre', *British Journal of Psychiatry*, August 1968.
4. Social Services Committee, *Community Care, Vol. 1: Report and Proceedings*, HMSO 1985, HC13-1.
5. Anthony Fry and P. W. Timms, 'Homeless and Rootless Action and Research Project Stage 2', unpublished paper.
6. Charlie Legg and Ada Kay, *Discharged into the Community*, City University 1984.
7. E. Baxter and K. Hopper, *Private Lives/Public Spaces*, Community Service Society (New York) 1981.
8. John A. Talbot et al., *The Homeless Mentally Ill*, The Amercian Psychiatric Task Force on the Homeless Mentally Ill.
9. Larry Gostin, 'America is no Haven for Mentally Ill People', *Social Work Today*, 15 December 1986.

10. Harry Reid and Alban Wiseman, *When the Talking has to Stop*, MIND Publications 1986.
11. Alison Wertheimer, *Hospital Closures in the Eighties*, The Campaign for People with Mental Handicaps 1986.
12. Ron Thomson, 'Dossing Down', *OPENMIND*, No. 15, June/July 1985.
13. Jane Ritchie and Jill Keegan, *Housing for Mentally Ill and Mentally Handicapped People*, HMSO 1983.
14. R. Eley and R. Middleton, 'Square Pegs, Round Holes', *Health Trends*, August 1983, p. 69.
15. Ritchie and Keegan, *Housing for Mentally Ill and Mentally Handicapped People*.

8

Therapeutic Communities – Halfway Home?

DR BOB GROVE

An evaluation of the therapeutic community in the care and management of people with mental problems at this time of mass unemployment and social division might seem almost an indulgence. In another time, when health care of all kinds is free to all according to need at the point of delivery, then the virtues, limitations and possibilities of the therapeutic community might make interesting discussion points. However, the United Kingdom in 1986 is as far from providing for even the most basic needs of a quarter of its population, whether or not they have mental health problems, that any discussion of a concept which assumes a comfortable standard of housing, nutrition, warmth, clothing and paid employment as the next stage of life, must be seen as an investment for better days to come.

This chapter will, therefore, sketch in the history and practice of the therapeutic community and attempt some kind of evaluation of the way the concept has developed. In common with all other discussions of how society should respond to people with mental health problems, the central questions revolve around the nature of the power relationships between those who have come to be designated as ill, and those who have taken on the roles of carer and healer. I shall argue that the pioneers of the therapeutic community concept tended to avoid such issues by developing an ideology which emphasized insight and self-awareness and assumed adjustment to the social norms of the carers. None the less the opportunity for member participation in the running of the communities was a valued innovation and, for many people, membership of a therapeutic community, a small but significant step on the road to self-confidence and independence.

Early Developments

Since the 1920s and 1930s, sociologists, psychiatrists and social psychologists have at various times and in various places challenged the notion of mental illness as a pathological malfunction of the individual psyche. Laing,[1] Scheff,[2] Maxwell Jones[3] and others focused attention on the individual's relationship to his or her social environment, both as a causal factor in precipitating breakdown, and as a potentially therapeutic factor in recovery and rehabilitation. Practitioners of 'milieu therapy' have always been a minority within the fields of psychiatry and social education, but their influence (and notoriety) has extended gradually into the mainstream of psychiatric and social work practice to the extent that the term 'therapeutic community' is now well known, if not well understood.

From the end of the Second World War, when Bion and Main[4] set up the Northfields Experiment, Birmingham and Maxwell Jones began the Belmont Rehabilitation Unit, Sutton, Surrey, the development of the therapeutic community has been almost wholly based within a psychiatric framework and the communities themselves have very frequently been located within the grounds of mental hospitals. This is unsurprising since the pioneers were all psychiatrists and, although critical of the heavy reliance of mainstream psychiatry on medication and ECT, only Laing ever wholly rejected the power structure of doctor/patient relationship, and the segregation of patients from the rest of the community through hospitalization.

The first therapeutic communities were designed for people who had broken down in wartime (Northfields), or had found difficulty in coping with the transition back to civilian life (Belmont). The central feature of the philosophy was the sharing of problems and insights into one's own and other people's behaviour, and the maintenance of caring attitudes and high group morale.

As with psychoanalysis, the emphasis was on 'talk-therapy' and, indeed, some of the innovators made considerable use of their analytic background in the daily community and group meetings. There is, however, a crucial difference between the therapeutic community and the psycho-therapeutic group, in that the community lives and works together, and therefore behaviour and relationships are constantly under scrutiny. Maxwell Jones referred to the Belmont (later the Henderson) as a 'living-learning' community and to the process as 'social learning'.[5] His was a classic 'self-adjustment' model of treatment which emphasized conformity to accepted social norms.

In a sociological study of the Henderson, Rapoport[6] identified four concepts which are of major ideological significance to staff working in therapeutic communities: (1) democratization; (2) permissiveness; (3) communalism; (4) reality confrontation. The exact meaning of these slogans is specific to the institutions, and Rapoport describes at some length the difficulties, contradictions and qualifications which the staff indicated in their replies to the value questionnaire he administered. Democratization, for instance, is not to be equated with political democracy, and permissiveness certainly does not imply sexual licence. The terms can best be understood in relation to the changing forms of social organization and social control in the conventional mental hospitals of the time.

Thus, democratization refers to the desirability of patients and staff participating in some degree of decision-making in the unit, rather than having decisions imposed on them as 'doctors' orders'. The rationale for this was that patients' negative feelings towards authority should be defused, and their own talents for helping each other, for leadership and for creativity, stimulated.

Communalism does not mean that staff and patients should live together in a commune, but rather that staff should participate with patients in domestic tasks, meals and leisure activities, so that the therapeutic potential of all aspects of life should be utilized. Thus the division of labour in a conventional hospital – its hierarchy of tasks and grades of worker with the patient either passive or allowed to help only with the most menial tasks – is broken down to a certain degree (theoretically a patient could be helping a consultant to clean the toilets).

Permissiveness simply means the toleration of a greater degree of behavioural licence than in most mental hospitals, before physical or chemical restraint is applied.

Reality confrontation refers to the belief that patients should be continuously presented with interpretations and the consequences of their behaviour as they are seen by others in the community. This is partly negotiated within the group, and partly a conscious attempt to confront patients with the social attitudes and conditions they will meet outside the community.

The lack of precision and definitional clarity about these principles was not regarded by the staff as unhelpful or antitherapeutic; quite the reverse. It was the continuous discussion about how far someone should be allowed to transgress before the community stepped in to set limits, as well as who should make decisions and above all the dialogue about the quality of commitment to the community and the therapeutic process, which were seen as maintaining the psychic and dynamic life of the community. Rapoport, however, pointed to the dangers both of the staff presenting their middle-class values as 'reality' to patients from other social backgrounds, and of the staff's failure to distinguish between treatment and rehabilitation or, as he puts it, between 'the alteration of the individual personality towards better intra-psychic integration' and 'the fitting of a particular personality to the demands of an ongoing social system'.

The need to maintain professional respectability and control over the 'acting out' behaviour of the patients has led to a whole range of self-justificatory ideologies which serve to manipulate and reduce the choices available to patients to what is broadly acceptable to the professionals and the wider public. These constraints apply to all social work and medical practice, but in a therapeutic community they are felt to be particularly acute because of the continuous discussion of the limits of acceptable behaviour, and the relentless scrutiny of the decision-making process. The hospital setting and the medically-trained staff provide, in many ways, a less constrained environment for experimentation. The hospital as an institution provides privacy and medical authority for practices which can there be labelled 'treatment' (but which elsewhere might be considered dangerous), or for perhaps condoning anti-social, even criminal, behaviour. The licence to speak freely the unspeakable seems only acceptable in the privacy of a consulting room, or the environs of an insane asylum ...

Outside the Hospital

Experiments with therapeutic communities outside hospitals have, therefore, never been widespread and have frequently been surrounded with controversy. Laing's early work at Kingsley Hall drew much criticism from professionals and the public, mostly because of the apparent licence to produce 'mad' behaviour in close proximity to those who liked to think of themselves as sane.

Only one organization has developed, in any systematic way, the 'halfway house' therapeutic community outside the hospital. The Richmond Fellowship, a charity founded in 1959 by Elly Jansen,[7] a Dutch nurse and theology student, has now set up 40 or more therapeutic communities of different sizes and for different client groups in the UK, and a similar number abroad.

Elly Jansen's experiment began at much the same time as Laing, Clark,[8] Maxwell Jones, Crockett[9] and others were trying to establish the therapeutic community as a major part of hospital treatment for people with mental health problems. The effects of the revolution in psychotropic medication and the 'open door' policies of the major mental hospitals had shortened the time people were expected to stay in hospital, and there was a new emphasis on cure, rather than containment. Jansen saw, however, that for most people leaving hospital, the preparation and after-care was minimal, and that the inadequacies in their personal relationships, and the total loss of confidence in themselves which inevitably follow mental breakdown, made it highly likely that they would quickly break down again. Renting a house in Richmond at her own expense, she put up notices in the local mental hospitals inviting people who were about to leave, to join her in a community dedicated to learning and mutual support. It was a brave and essentially pragmatic experiment which encountered fierce resistance from the professional establishment, both on the grounds of her lack of professional qualifications, and mainly for her insistence that people recovering from a mental breakdown should learn to rejoin the wider community by actually living there.

Over the years, the doubters were persuaded or lost interest and the Fellowship now has a certain respectability – indeed, in some quarters, a reputation for conservatism and stuffiness which would have been most surprising to the first (very few) supporters of Jansen's pioneering work. None the less, a solid body of experience has been built up over the years which forms the basis not only of a number of different and quite specialized forms of therapeutic community, but also of a staff training programme in therapeutic community work, which is still unique.

Living in a Therapeutic Community

The patterns of daily life vary from community to community, depending on the needs and age of the residents, the number (between ten and 50), and the culture which has developed. A house for people who have been diagnosed as suffering from chronic schizophrenia, and for whom it is likely to be home for a long time, will have very few formal meetings – a community meeting once a week, plus a Saturday morning clean-up – and the residents will be encouraged to find work or day-time activities outside.

On the other hand, a house where people are in need of a short period of rehabilitation may have a semi-formal group each morning, and weekly small groups in addition to the weekly community meeting. Leisure activities may be structured to fill most afternoons, and the staff will meet frequently to analyse the dynamics and morale of the community and work on inter-staff relationships.

Such intense scrutiny of feelings and relationships can lead to a highly emotionally charged atmosphere and an acute sensitivity to apparently minor events. The mood of the whole community can swing abruptly when a key member leaves, or a new person comes in. A minor piece of delinquency can plunge the community into deep depression or anger which pervades the whole group, and it is the work of the staff to lead the group through such experiences to a resolution. The rationale for creating this highly charged environment is that, having helped people to excavate the feelings behind self-destructive behavioural patterns, the shared work of the group will teach new strategies for dealing with the feelings, and more acceptable ways of behaving.

The staff are not immune to the prevailing emotional climate and spend much time away from the community working on their own anger and depression. They also plan strategies for manipulating the social environment of the community in order to achieve an acceptable balance between permissiveness and social control, both for themselves and for the wider community.

The Community Meeting

Central to the process of all therapeutic communities is the community meeting. The whole community will meet daily, or at least weekly, to discuss anything from the practicalities of running the house, to a delinquent episode which has upset or disturbed the community. In some communities there is an agenda prepared by staff and for residents in which a period of unstructured discussion may be permitted. In others there is no agenda, and subjects for discussion are allowed to rise to the surface, theoretically enabling the skilled staff member or experienced resident to detect the main anxieties or dynamics and facilitate discussion.

There are also variations in the objectives of discussion. In a comparative study of two communities,[10] I found a considerable contrast between the community meeting, where the focus was almost wholly on pushing the individuals to consider their motivations and the feelings behind particular forms of behaviour, and another style of meeting, where the object seemed to be principally to exert group pressure on the individual to behave differently. In the former, a psychotherapeutic ideology was very deeply embedded in the life of the community, giving priority to insight and self-knowledge, whereas in the latter the emphasis was almost wholly on task performance and producing socially acceptable behaviour. The Richmond Fellowship model certainly favours the latter approach though there is at best a sharing of feelings and a degree of compassion, which to some people makes the therapeutic community a particularly acceptable way of dealing with mental and emotional problems.

The following extract from a community meeting in a half-way house illustrates both the pressures to conform, and the sharing of painful feelings. Penny[11] has been slashing her arms to the distress of other residents. There has been some discussion of this in a small group meeting, and Tom* is reporting back.

Tom*: ... and then Penny did most of the talking. I was asking her about her agreement which she was going to talk to the community about – as I understand it, going back some days now – chiefly about cutting her arms. And Penny spoke about being not sure whether she really wished herself to do this, or really felt under a sort of compulsion to make the agreement.

Helen: Any feedback?

William: Are you going to make this agreement tonight Penny?

Penny: Yes ...

Later towards the end of the meeting.

Helen: Well, Penny, it's time for your agreement.

Penny: Could we leave it till tomorrow?

Ann*: I'm not happy about you leaving it for another day.

Penny: Alright, I'll read it from the paper: go to all compulsory groups; not harm myself; try to talk to people when I get desperate; and eat lunch or supper every weekday with the community – at least one meal every weekday.

William: Sorry, what was the last bit?

Penny: Eating one meal with the community each weekday.

Tom*: And this is an agreement that, although you may have some ambivalent views about, you are saying please support me in this.

Penny: I suppose so.

Mary*: Which will be the hardest bit?

Penny: Talking to people instead of running away.

Mary*: That's the hardest bit, why?

Penny: Because I'm not used to showing my feelings. I'm not very honest about my feelings. I'm honest about things I've done, but not about my feelings.

William: Do you feel this house is getting you down, more and more depressed?

Penny: I'm getting more and more depressed.

William: Do you know why?

Penny: No, I'm getting more lonely, or at least I'm feeling it more.

William: I can understand how Penny feels actually. She's a very bright, bouncy member of the community, but she's very lonely inside. I get like that sometimes. I can sympathize with you.

Penny: Thanks.

William: (laughs) Don't know how to overcome it, but I can sympathize with you.

Evaluation

This account of the therapeutic community demonstrates both the virtues and limitations of the concept. It does provide an opportunity for people to live in a situation in which there is help available in learning to sustain personal relationships prior to returning to permanent or semi-permanent domestic arrangements. For some, the larger community is more congenial than small 'family-size' domestic units, especially when their own family lives have contributed largely to their trauma.

For these benefits, however, there is a price to be paid in restrictions on individual choice of action and lifestyle, and also in the reproduction in that particular setting of the structured power relationships between the 'ill' and the 'well' – the medical model in another disguise?

Other objections to the therapeutic community have been made on the basis that because the ideology requires some ability to conceptualize and articulate feelings and experiences, it can only be effective for people with a relatively high level of intellectual and educational development. And, indeed, in both small communities I used for my research, the residents were overwhelmingly white and middle class, with a much higher than average level of educational attainment. As with many other aspects of the therapeutic community, no large-scale research work has been done, and so those who would criticize are left with their impressions and their prejudices. However, one thing that all workers in the mental health field agree on, is that there must be a range of provisions to suit different needs.

A far more central question is whether or not the therapeutic community achieves its objectives; that is, does it enable people to gain or recover the ability to live satisfactory lives outside hospital? Once again, there is a dearth of research information. This is not solely due to the unwillingness on the part of practitioners to have their work subjected to scrutiny. It is difficult to draw up any but the most crude criteria of success and failure. Rates of readmission to hospital might be a guide, but not necessarily an indication of the quality of life achieved by those who are not readmitted. Impressive figures showing few readmissions may indicate more about the changing policy of the health authority than the mental state of former patients etc.

There is a further problem, in that once having agreed criteria of success and failure, it is very difficult indeed to establish whether the results for any individual are attributable to any part of the community programme.

Those who are critical of the therapeutic community claim that the skills it teaches are not those that ensure survival outside; that the community is in fact a subtle form of institutionalization where people learn only how to survive in that particular environment. Certainly, the evidence from my own work suggests that the ability of staff to manipulate the social environment is matched by an increased tendency among residents to develop coping strategies which, at times, bear a close resemblance to the sub-culture of more obviously institutional environments.

On the other hand, those who have worked in therapeutic communities would say that over a longer period of time, a community oscillates between rigidity and flexibility and that some people experience, perhaps for the first time, a real inner freedom in their social relationships. Practitioners can point to case histories where a person's self-confidence and social skills have improved dramatically and permanently during a period within a therapeutic community. Some report that residents who have left, and for whom the therapeutic environment was an apparent failure, return in later years to claim that, in the long term, the experience was the turning point in their lives. Such evidence is anecdotal, but cannot be dismissed entirely, especially when there is equally little evidence that any other route towards mental health is likely to produce better results.

Conclusion

It is my view that the verdict on the therapeutic community is, and will remain, 'case unproven'. But whether or not the therapeutic community concept develops will not depend on what at any given time people regard as success or failure, but on society's response to mental health problems, which in turn is determined by economic, political and moral considerations. That response, in terms of government support, has been extremely poor; the gross under-funding of care in the community, and the housing crisis which is denying to many who have long-term mental health problems even a roof over their heads, are problems which, unless resolved, will subvert all attempts to improve mental health care in this country.

Meanwhile the current ideological debate between those who advocate 'normalization' in housing and community care, and those who see virtues in continuing hospital-type care, has tended to marginalize discussion of the therapeutic community as a halfway house. This is not necessarily unhealthy, since it leaves the people who want to set up and develop these practical services, to get on with the job without incurring much negative attention from either ideological camp.

Clearly, the therapeutic community is not, in its original conception, a suitable form of long-term housing for people with long-term mental health problems. But as part of a process of rehabilitation, it is arguably very successful for some people.

The major contribution of the therapeutic community movement has been its stance against the complete medicalization of mental health problems, and its demonstration that a social environment which emphasizes participation and constructive dialogue about personal relationships can be extremely valuable as a way of easing the isolation and loss of confidence which come with the onset of mental breakdown. The latter is, of course, a principle which should be central to all forms of community care and it is no small achievement by those who have pioneered therapeutic communities that this is now becoming received wisdom.

Notes

1. R. D. Laing, *The Divided Self*, Tavistock 1960.
2. T. J. Scheff, *Being Mentally Ill*, Weidenfeld and Nicolson 1966.
3. M. Jones, *Social Psychiatry*, Tavistock 1952.
4. T. Main, 'The Hospital as a Therapeutic Institution', *Bulletin of the Meninger Clinic*, No. 10, 1946, p. 66.
5. Jones, *Social Psychiatry*.
6. R. Rapoport, *Community As Doctor*, Tavistock 1960.
7. E. Jansen, *The Therapeutic Community Outside The Hospital*, Croom Helm 1980.
8. D. H. Clark, *Administrative Therapy*, Tavistock 1964.
9. R. Crockett, 'Doctor, Administrator and the Therapeutic Community', *The Lancet*, No. 2, 1960, pp. 359–63.
10. R. Grove, 'Negotiation and Social Order in the Therapeutic Community', unpublished PhD thesis, 1985.
11. All names have been changed; staff members are identified by an asterisk after the name.

Private Enterprise in the Care Vacuum

ALISON NORMAN

In a damning critique of the failure of community care, the government's own Audit Commission said in 1986,

> Over 300,000 people live in residential settings. The reduction of NHS facilities has been offset by the growth in private residential homes where some residents are entitled to receive help with their fees from supplementary benefit. In 1984 some 40,000 residents were receiving such help at a cost of some £200 million; but the Commission estimates that the cost is now £500 million a year and growing rapidly. At best there seems to be a shift from one pattern of residential care based on hospitals to an alternative supported in many cases by supplementary benefit payments – missing out more flexible and cost-effective forms of community care altogether ... Meanwhile, local authorities are often penalized through the grant system for building up the very community services which government policy favours and which are necessary if the NHS is to close its large long-stay hospitals.[1]

That is the position in a nutshell. The current explosion in the numbers of very old people (there will be an increase of nearly a million people aged 75 or more between 1981 and the end of the century), combined with the drive to close long-stay hospitals for both mentally distressed and mentally handicapped people, has created a demand for appropriate housing and support services which is not being met by the local authorities. The private sector has stepped into that yawning vacuum of care, but control over the appropriateness of the care which it offers is minimal. At one extreme, public money is being poured out to provide over-protective care for people who could lead fairly independent lives, and at the other, supplementary benefit rates are insufficient to buy proper care for very disabled people. In short, the most vulnerable members of our society are at the receiving end of a total mess.

A few figures illustrate the speed of growth.

Non-statutory Homes and Hostels 1975 and 1985 (England)				
	No. of Homes		No. of Places	
	1975	1985	1975	1985
Mental Illness				
Private	26	102	472	1,219
Voluntary	41	148	894	1,952
Total	67	250	1,366	3,171
Mental Handicap				
Private	73	231	1,101	3,105
Voluntary	56	232	1,784	3,991
Total	129	463	2,885	7,096
Elderly				
Private	1,770	5,200	24,606	80,041
Voluntary	1,091	1,108	33,319	37,466
Total	2,861	6,308	57,925	117,507

Sources: Weekly Hansard 1392, 21–5 July 1986. Health and Personal Social Services Statistics for England, HMSO 1986.

In the fields of both mental handicap and mental illness, the private sector has trebled the number of places it provides during the last ten years and is fast catching up on the voluntary sector, though that too has greatly expanded. In both cases, the increase in the number of homes is considerably greater than the increase in the number of beds. This drop in the average size of home is particularly noticeable in the voluntary mental handicap homes – reflecting the new philosophy of service provision.

In the much larger field of provision for elderly people (including a small number of places for people with physical handicaps), the voluntary sector has remained almost static in the number of homes it provides, although the average size of home has increased somewhat. In the private sector, however, the number of both homes and places has again trebled, but from a very much larger base, and is now over twice the size of the voluntary sector and four-fifths of the total for local authority homes.

It is worth looking briefly at how this situation has come about.[2] Until 1980 very few people were in private care unless they could afford to pay the fees themselves. However, local authorities made extensive use of the voluntary sector to house people for whom they themselves could not provide suitable care. The level of fees charged was agreed between the voluntary organization concerned and the local authority in which the home was situated, and this agreement was accepted by other authorities which used the home. (A similar arrangement could be made with a private proprietor, but this was rare except in the case of nursing home beds contracted to the NHS.) People with limited resources could be 'sponsored' by the local authority – that is the local authority would make up the shortfall between what the person was deemed to be able to afford and the full charge. In general, however, the social services departments did not consider themselves to have responsibility for arranging care for people with severe dependency needs and the NHS provided long-stay hospital care for a very large number of people with mental handicap, mental health problems or chronic physical disability.

In 1980 a crucial piece of legislation relating to supplementary benefit regulations made it clear that the board and lodging allowance, which had previously been payable to people living in hotels and boarding houses on a commercial basis, could also be used to pay charges in residential care homes and nursing homes. For the first time an individual could obtain private care without either assessment of need or a private income, and private care became one of the country's few growth industries. This was not, by and large, the result of wealthy entrepreneurs jumping in to make a cynical and exploitative fortune, although some big concerns are now getting into the market. Many of the new proprietors were owners of guest houses and small seaside hotels who had lost their trade to the Costa del Sol and welcomed the idea of permanent guests backed by government funds. Other new proprietors were looking for a way of investing redundancy pay in a business which would provide accommodation, income and freedom from the fear of the sack. Many nurses felt that they could make more effective use of their skills and get a more reasonable income by running a nursing home than by slaving for a pittance in the NHS.

The resultant explosion in costs to the DHSS rapidly convinced the government that it must set limits to the open-ended discretionary powers of the local DHSS offices to pay fees, and in November 1983 it introduced a new three-tier system whereby locally determined maximum limits were set for three categories of accommodation: ordinary board and lodging, residential care homes and nursing homes. The revised limits were set at a level which reflected the highest 'reasonable' charge for suitable accommodation in the area. This resulted in very wide variations in local limits – ranging from £51 a week to £215 a week in residential care homes – and it encouraged home owners who had been charging below the limits to raise their fees to the maximum allowed. Far from limiting costs, therefore, they rose from £39 million in 1982 to nearly £200 million in 1985. In 1985, in a further attempt to check the escalation, it was announced that individuals in residential care homes were to be divided into categories depending on the nature of their handicap and a national limit of charges met by the DHSS set for each category. An additional amount was payable to nursing homes and hospices but the attendance allowance was not, as hitherto, excluded from the calculation. People who were already in care were allowed to continue to receive benefit at the previous rate, but this was not increased if fees went up.

This system, which is still in force, has a number of serious drawbacks.

• It deliberately discriminates against elderly citizens. People suffering from mental handicap, mental disorder or physical handicap who are under pensionable age receive a higher allowance than residents in non-specialist old people's homes no matter how severely disabled they are. Moreover, although local authorities are permitted to help with charges higher than the national limit by 'topping up' the supplementary benefit rates for younger residents, they are not allowed to do so for elderly people unless they were severely dependent before reaching pensionable age.

- The limits set (even with subsequent upratings) are not sufficient to cover the cost of providing 24-hour care for very dependent people, but they are over-generous with regard to people who simply need 'protection' and crisis care.
- The limits are set on a national basis with no consideration of local and regional variations in cost.
- There is an assumption that local authorities will 'top up' as required for dependent younger people, but with government squeezes on their expenditure, this is very often not the case.

The government has not even succeeded in its attempt to apply uniform procedures across the country. There is confusion as to what types of 'high care' accommodation qualify for the higher residential care home rate.

In addition to attempting to set limits on the cost of providing non-statutory care, the government also attempted to ensure that care was provided to an adequate standard. The Registered Homes Act 1984 gave health and social services authorities extensive powers and duties in the registration and regular inspection of residential homes and nursing homes. They can refuse or withdraw registration if standards are not satisfactory, subject to an appeal to a tribunal. With the Act was published a Code of Practice[3] which sets out in some detail the principles of good care by which the proprietors and the inspecting authorities should be guided. There were however at least six main failings in the legislation.

1. It set registration fees at a level which was insufficient to pay

for a proper system of registration, advice-giving and inspection.

2. It only covered establishments which provided care for four or more people. 'Cottage industry' care is still totally unregulated. (This is now a very considerable branch of the market, though by definition no one knows how large it is. Ralph Chapman, East Sussex Chief Registration Officer, estimates that there are about 300 such establishments in East Sussex alone.) One serious consequence of this loophole is that proprietors who have had their registration withdrawn because of malpractice can continue to operate with three clients.

3. It perpetuated the anomalous and nonsensical distinction between nursing care and personal care which dates back to the National Assistance Act 1948. (Private nursing homes, which are registered by the health authorities, have their own, very different code of practice which puts less emphasis on privacy and quality of life and more on professional qualifications of staff and nursing procedures.)

4. It failed to set up a central monitoring inspectorate which would ensure that local authorities and health authorities carried out their duties under the Act in a conscientious and reasonably uniform way. In consequence, some authorities seem to be doing an excellent job while others are making much more extensive demands than the Act or the Code of Practice require, or are interpreting the regulations in an inflexible and pettifogging way. Many have not yet 'got their act together' or are deliberately turning a blind eye to bad practice – often in the knowledge that the homes which they themselves run are even worse. Over-rigid interpretation of the law can itself help to create an institutional atmosphere and result in inappropriate levels of staffing or selection of staff so that the opportunity for relatively independent and 'normal' living is reduced. The Code of Practice emphasizes that its general guidelines need to be interpreted in the light of the aims of particular establishments, but this is not always attempted, let alone achieved.

5. The Act gave local authorities no power to deal with the owners of boarding houses who deliberately cram their rooms with highly vulnerable people with a history of alcoholism or mental health problems but who then make no claim to provide the extra support which is needed and so are not required to apply for registration as a residential care home.

6. The system of appeal to a tribunal has proved to be lengthy and expensive especially when appellants hire top-class lawyers. This means that authorities may be over-cautious in the exercise of their powers, and 'borderline' homes are allowed to continue to function. Furthermore, the membership of each tribunal is different and they vary in their views of the way in which the Act should be applied, so that no standard 'case law' is built up.

In spite of these disadvantages, the Act seems to be working reasonably well in ensuring the quality of care in new establishments, provided it is applied by well-trained staff of sufficient numbers and status. It is, however, much more difficult to ensure that standards are maintained in homes which have been operating for a number of years, and where staff and proprietor may themselves have become 'institutionalized'. This danger applies with even greater force to the voluntary sector. Long-established voluntary bodies set up to provide care – which may well have been excellent for its day – may now have utterly un-suitable facilities and an outdated paternalistic approach to their task. In this situation, it is not easy for a registration officer to apply the same standards as he would with a new home in the private sector – the more so if a religious order is involved or, as in the case of local Mencap societies, if it is the parents of the handicapped people who have outdated concepts of what 'care' should be like.

The registration of homes catering for people with a chronic mental disablement or mental handicap raises other complex issues. For example, if a local authority is itself setting up family-sized groups in ordinary housing for these clients, it seems illogical to accept applications for larger and more institutional units from the private sector. However, neither the Registered Homes Act nor the Code of Practice lays down any rules in this regard, and it is not clear what authority officers have to refuse registration on these grounds alone. East Sussex recently refused to allow a home to increase its registration from six to nine residents because this would reduce the 'homeliness' of the establishment, while in North Wales in 1986 a tribunal only decided by 2–1 that a colony of mentally handicapped adults should not be permitted to raise its registration from 107 to 124 residents.

Another problem is that there is no clear demarcation line between 'care' and 'protection' for people who are temporarily or minimally disabled – what may matter is that help should be available in times of crisis or regression rather than having it imposed whether it is needed or not. Does such support constitute 'care' under the Act?

There is also the matter of responsibility to provide day-time activity. Some authorities refuse to register new homes which accept residents from outside the county unless proprietors can show that they are providing suitable activity with properly qualified staff outside the residential establishment and that the situation of the home enables residents to make full use of ordinary community and commercial facilities. They are not, they say, 'in the business of re-creating the total institution'. (As a result, some proprietors have become specialists in this field and 'sell' day places to other home owners so that day-care is becoming an industry in its own right.) However, many authorities do not ensure that adequate facilities for day-time occupation are provided or available.

'Mix' of disability is another difficult area. Proprietors who accept residents of all degrees of disability can 'trade off' the heavy staffing needs of profoundly handicapped people against the minimal care required by the others and so keep their fees within the supplementary benefit limits. This does not create optimum conditions for less disabled residents. More able residents may also not be sufficiently encouraged to acquire skills in cooking and housework for fear of charges of 'exploitation'.

A further issue arises over the concentration of homes for particular areas. East Sussex, for example, has for many years been a source of placements for care – a tradition which first developed because of the facilities offered by the Brighton Guardianship Society and which then spread to other homes. Considerable numbers of residents are placed in private or voluntary care in the county by some of the London Boroughs and by adjoining authorities.

This practice gives rise to a number of complications. For example, the distance from the resident's original home means that contact with both family and the responsible social worker is likely to be minimal, and there will be little active support in working towards a less protective environment. Also in some cases the 'out-county' authority may disagree with the responsible registration officer about the quality of care offered in an establishment. It has been known for proprietors accused of mistreatment of residents to defend themselves by calling evidence from social workers in other authorities whose concepts of 'care' differ from the registering authority. In some areas, planning departments have attempted to prevent further 'importation' of residents by refusing permission for new homes on general environmental grounds, but this is of doubtful legal validity and also has the effect of artificially increasing the value of existing homes.

The situation is thus difficult and complex for the local authorities, the health authorities and the local DHSS officers, but it is also by no means easy for proprietors who at times are being asked to provide greatly improved standards of care and accommodation, plus a large increase in registration costs, in a situation where fees payable from supplementary benefit bear no relationship to the dependency of residents. Very often also, proprietors have incurred a heavy capital debt when setting up the home and have borrowed the money assuming that the original system of setting the level of fees paid by supplementary benefit would continue. That debt has to be repaid and serviced. Under the present fee-paying system, the proprietor has to choose between refusing residents who need a lot of care so that he or she can cut down on staffing costs, and refusing residents who cannot find a means of 'topping up' their fees above supplementary benefit level. But he or she also has to keep beds full and this is most easily done by accepting patients who would otherwise be candidates for long-stay hospital care and who are dependent on supplementary benefit. Low staffing and high dependency inevitably lead to poor care – 'care of the orifices' as one informant described it. Thus, yet again, people who are most poor, most disadvantaged and most at risk, lose out.

All this confusion has been worse compounded by the government's desire to push through its policy of closing the old psychiatric hospitals and mental handicap hospitals in which many people with various degrees of disability have lived for many years. There is very strong pressure on hospital management to clear beds and if good private care is available there is a strong temptation to grab the places – using 'care in the community' 'dowries' to top up fees above supplementary benefit levels if necessary – and without proper assessment as to whether the individuals concerned really require that sort of care.[4] For example, the *Health Service Journal* reports that Frenchay Health Authority (Bristol) paid £50,000 in advance to a private nursing home to care for two dependent mentally handicapped patients over a five-year period – in addition to the supplementary benefit payment of £190 a week to which the patients were entitled. It was claimed that this arrangement would save the health authority at least £6,000 a year.[5] Such money goes down the drain – it does nothing to fund a proper alternative source of care which will outlive the patients concerned.

Often the nurses who have been caring for particular individuals in hospital will set up a nursing home and apply to take over 'their' patients. Alternatively, nurses may buy residential property near a psychiatric hospital which is due for closure and persuade patients to come and live with them with a view to using their benefit to pay off the mortgage and on the assumption that the ex-patients will be out all day at the hospital's day facilities. If the hospital no longer provides this facility or the landlady has made enough money to meet the mortgage repayments, such ex-patients are liable to find themselves homeless and without social-work protection.

There is also gross exploitation of homeless single people – often ex-psychiatric hospital patients – in overcrowded substandard lodging houses. The environmental health authorities may be powerless to prosecute because they cannot identify the responsible person[6] and, as was noted above, no action can be taken under the registration system if there is no claim to provide care – however much that care may be needed. Inevitably, where there are landlords looking for lodgers and homeless ex-patients looking for somewhere to live, the two are going to meet up and the lodger in that situation is wide open to exploitation.

Given the confusion and the insecurity of hospital care, it is not surprising that anxious parents of mentally handicapped people are pressing for hospital sites to be re-vamped as 'village communities' for mentally handicapped people – a solution which the enthusiasts for 'normalization' simply see as the old hospital system under another name.[7] (They are almost equally unenthusiastic about schemes whereby a housing association or other voluntary organization agrees to house former long-stay patients and a health authority promises to top up fees and provide nursing and medical services. In some of these arrangements there is a wholesale transfer of hospital-trained staff and medical control so that the 'medical model' of long-term care is perpetuated.)

As the Audit Commission's report quoted above says,

If nothing changes, the outlook is bleak … the opportunity for building a community-based service will not remain open indefinitely: once an alternative service based on residential homes is in place, vested interests and institutional inertia can be expected to block any major changes in patterns of care.

Notes
1. *Making a Reality of Community Care: a Report by the Audit Commission*, HMSO 1986.

2. Detailed information about these changes and their consequences is provided by Christine Peaker, *The Crisis in Residential Care*, National Council for Voluntary Organisations 1986.
3. *Home Life: A Code of Practice for Residential Care*, Centre for Policy on Ageing 1984.
4. L. Hoyes and L. Harrison, 'An Ordinary Life or Imitation?', *Community Care*, 12 February 1987.
5. *Health Service Journal*, 6 March 1986.
6. Monica Brimacombe, 'Dumping the mentally ill', *Roof*, November/December 1986 (with an untitled follow-up in the January/February issue).
7. Boyd Tonkin, 'Voices in the Wilderness', *Community Care*, 15 January 1987.

10

The Poor Laws Revisited

CATHERINE GRIMSHAW

> People do not go on to social security to escape poverty. Living just on social security is poverty. But social security is more than just a question of money. It is also a question of how people are treated, about the kind of reception they get and the pressures to which they are subjected. – Tony Novak[1]

Poverty has many faces and as many disguises. Patients in a long-stay psychiatric ward who have their immediate needs for food, warmth and shelter met by the hospital, can lead lives just as impoverished as those who make their home from a cardboard box under the stars. For behind the trappings of people's existence lies their fundamental need for a regular, accessible and adequate amount of income in order to participate in the life of the community. If that need remains unrecognized or unmet, then any 'home', however constituted, becomes a prison. Within that prison you may not be starved of basic necessities but you will certainly be starved of choice.

However, to be poor is not only to live without enough money; it is to experience a profound sense of ostracism by a culture that judges its citizens in terms of their wealth and the distance they can put between themselves and dependence on state assistance. 'Getting the state off people's backs' is an oft-quoted dictum of 'laissez-faire' philosophy. The state is restrictive and commonly seen as an obstacle to progress rather than as an aid – that is if you have the resources and can look after yourself. Self-reliance combined with a competitive spirit are therefore praised and encouraged as the perfect character traits which lead to success, i.e. riches. To rely on the state for financial support is seen as shameful; it is proof that you have 'failed' and are 'out of the race'.

Work is what all this is about, because work does not only supply an independent source of income, it also confers self-esteem and an acknowledged position in society upon the worker. The more prestigious the job, the greater the status. We are surrounded by the image – and its endless variations – of the successful businessman who, as a result of his employment and the distinction it carries, is also invited to select the rewards that accompany success: the sleek company car, the bountiful credit card and the glamorous companion.

For those of us who are able to partake of the fruits of our affluent society, life may be relatively untouched by the plight of those who cannot. Indeed, many people express indignation at footing the cost of running a system of state income support for those whose ability to earn sufficient sums is impaired. 'In a few short years the ground has shifted so decisively that in-equality is not only accepted by many people as inevitable but has acquired a Thatcherite tingle of merit for keeping us on our toes.'[2] Interwoven in our culture is the notion that by dint of hard labour and personal thrift you cannot fail to prosper. And those people who do not prosper have only themselves to blame – they are too lazy to work or find themselves a better job, or they are too irresponsible to budget, so it is their fault they exclude themselves from the rewards our society puts on offer to those who 'deserve' them.

How, then, does this society meet the needs of its citizens who, as a result of a disabling mental condition, are incapable of earning an independent income through employment, or who are unable to bear the extra financial costs that accompany poor mental health? And what is it like, given our judgemental culture, to be forced to rely on the state's 'safety net' – the social security system – to escape destitution? The answers to these questions are important, for already living in the community are significant numbers of the population with, or likely to develop, the symptoms we commonly term 'mental illness'.

Imagine you are unfortunate enough to be in such acute

mental distress that you can no longer continue in your job. In the first instance, you may be able to survive financially for a while on your occupational sick pay. Eventually, however, if your mental health deteriorates to such an extent that you become incapable of returning to paid work, then state assistance in the form of social security benefits will be the likely alternative to a salary.

At that stage, it is not just your source of income that has disappeared. Your self-esteem will have suffered as well. In short, your power to dictate your own lifestyle has been taken away. Like those people who have never worked, or only intermittently, because of their mental condition, your outlook for the future is not rosy. The features of mental ill-health may be hard enough to endure; coping with the prejudice and stigma that inevitably attend it is yet another struggle. Our fear and lack of acceptance of other people's behaviour, especially those who are labelled 'mad', and our disregard for their potential to work, if necessary with help and support, contributes to this process of devaluation – a process that both excludes the 'devalued' from a dignified role in the community, and at the same time offers no sanctuary from the disruption that mental distress inflicts. Being at the bottom of the pile does not mean you can escape from the practices of those at the top.

As public attitudes towards what is described as mental illness are notoriously backward and difficult to change, are the assumptions that lie behind state income provision any more enlightened? The answer is no. People who must dip into the state's purse for their sole source of income, or to supplement insufficient resources, find the same mistrustful attitudes mirrored in the way state assistance is devised, administered and perceived. For those citizens who are defined as incapable of servicing society through their labour, the state has created and consistently promoted a system of support that will not only keep them poor financially, it will also ensure that being impoverished applies to all other aspects of their life as well.

From the introduction of the Poor Laws in Elizabethan times, to the present day, claiming 'poor relief' has never been an easy option. For it is entirely consistent with the way society judges its citizens in terms of their productive capacity that the business of claiming 'relief' from the state should be made as unpleasant and stigmatizing as possible. The process of devaluation is completed by obliging claimants to negotiate their way through a complicated social security system, and then expecting them to budget on an amount that barely stretches to cover daily requirements, let alone enables them to meet the extra cost of mental ill-health or to play a part in the community around them.

Cut off from the means of earning an adequate and independent income, there is little to stop poverty, with its attendant restrictions, dogging the lives of people already disadvantaged by the limitations that a disabling mental condition imposes. Arresting that decline takes more than lip service to the principles of a 'care in the community' policy: it requires a wholesale change in our attitudes towards incapacity to work and dependency on the state.

Loud and clear have come the calls to successive governments to strengthen their commitment to social security, and equally firm has been the resistance to such appeals. Our present administration in particular has shown a marked intransigence, preferring to pursue as far as possible an unregulated economy that enables fortune to smile on those who help themselves without recourse to the state. This government makes much of the democratic and 'open' nature of our society. Therefore, in the name of 'care in the community' – a doctrine all the major parties say they support – it should be possible to bring pressure to reform the worst features of government policy and practice, if sufficient numbers of claimants and their supporters mobilized to express their resistance. However, a government committed first and foremost to making profits will actively collude in negating its citizens who are unable to derive sufficient income from work.

Denying people status also denies them power. This government in particular has not sought to bridge the growing gulf between rich and poor. Rather, it seeks to fuel the negative opinions of the general population towards claimants by its own allegations of idleness and fecklessness directed at groups of social security recipients. By doing so, it bolsters public resentment to extending state income support further, and presents this unpopularity as justification for introducing more restrictions on the right to state benefits.

As mental health problems tend to remain 'hidden' – unlike physical disability which is more 'visible' – it is more difficult for claimants who fall in the former category to dodge the label 'undeserving', and the prejudice that goes with it. It is hardly surprising then that such claimants should regard the system of state income support as omnipotent, as it is so often buttressed both by the government and the strength of public opinion. In their eyes, the same system is becoming less accountable and less responsive to those who must depend upon it. This is not to deny that large numbers of claimants (and their advocates) have in the past made commendable and sometimes successful efforts to challenge and change our social security system. The point is, however, that the weight of the government's resistance to spending more on combating poverty means that any improvements to social security remain slow, piecemeal and insufficient.

Furthermore, claimants at the sharp end are relatively powerless to confront a system on which they so heavily depend. Exerting pressure effectively is just not possible when you are grappling with the often unpredictable nature of mental ill-health within an environment that has such unsympathetic views of people unable to support themselves through work. Once you are dubbed as 'mad', opportunities to express opinions that are taken seriously, or to do battle with the Department of Social Security, are few.

Promoting a 'care in the community' policy on the one hand, and denying people an adequate level of income on the other, is, however, a recipe for failure. For keeping the poor in poverty has been demonstrated as a cause and a consequence of mental and physical ill-health.[3] Debt problems and the difficulties of managing on a low budget feature prominently amongst the reasons why people are admitted into psychiatric hospitals.[4]

This financial burden on the NHS and health-related services far outweighs what it would cost to expand the social security budget and enable people to cope in their own homes.

Recent statistics also show that as unemployment and poverty have risen so have death and disease.[5] Such findings are consistent with past studies on the effects of deprivation. For example, the Report of the Working Group on Inequalities in Health (the Black Report) in 1979 made abundantly clear the link between poverty and ill-health. Its conclusions were that, whereas biological and cultural influences are important factors in the nation's health, the level of material prosperity amongst members of the population determines the standard of health enjoyed. The Working Group warned, '. . . a new attack on the forces of inequality has regrettably become necessary.'

That the government of the day had a crucial and vigorous role to play in redressing inequality was plain. Yet the impact of the Report, with its call for a redistribution and injection of resources within the health and associated services, was met with a cool reception from this government. The Secretary of State refused to endorse the findings and was critical of the additional expenditure needed to implement the Report's recommendations. Such a negative response sits uneasily amongst this government's commitment to promote a community care policy, but is more at home perhaps within its determination to 'roll back the frontiers of the state'.

So, here is the heart of the matter. Care in the community implies a process of re-valuing citizens called mentally ill. Of necessity this means narrowing the gap between those who have and those who have not, by actively promoting an anti-poverty strategy. Therefore, no government which is serious about closing hospitals can simply sit back, cut spending on state benefits and let market forces determine the shape of tomorrow's society. To pretend otherwise is like saying that survival of the fittest really translates as caring in the community. As the Bishop of Durham cautioned in his contribution to the House of Lords Debate on Social Security in November 1985:

Social investment cannot entirely wait upon economic development. Maybe we have to give up any notion of jam today in the hope of producing jam tomorrow. Surely, it will be dangerously socially divisive if we start trying to scrape off what little margarine there is on some very dry bread, which is all that people at present have.

The promised reforms to social security made subsequent to a series of public Reviews of the system held in 1984 failed to deliver the changes necessary to remedy its obvious shortcomings. From the start, the government made it clear that any recommended changes to the system of state income support could not be implemented if additional expenditure had to be incurred. The new scheme outlined in the Social Security Act 1986, the government maintained, would result in a simpler, 'better-targetted' system that would take us forward to the twenty-first century. Moreover, the government boasted of the 'special attention we give to disabled people in our proposals'.[6] These statements simply do not stand up to scrutiny. Fewer basic rights, more means-testing and less rather than more financial support is the result – particularly for those groups of claimants who used to qualify for extra financial help because of their special needs. In other words, instead of using the Reviews as an opportunity to strengthen the 'safety net' of social security for those claimants already vulnerable because of their mental condition, the government has deliberately weakened it. Why?

Brian Abel-Smith and Peter Townsend point out that, since the present government took office, it has greatly increased public expenditure on defence, law and order and on maintaining able-bodied people who are unable to find work, when, '... the extra cash ... could alternatively have been used to increase the levels of social security benefits of 1978 to 1979 by over 20 per cent. Instead ... social security is being made the scapegoat for the government's ill-chosen priorities and disastrous economic management.'[7] This government saw in the overhaul of social security the opportunity to save money regardless of the social and economic consequences of keeping large numbers of people on the poverty line. And despite intensive lobbying on the part of organizations of and for people with both mental and physical disabilities, and despite the merits of their case, their efforts made virtually no impact on the final shape of the Act.

Thus, the politics of invalidity teach us as much about the lengths a government can and will go to to escape the legitimate concerns of its less privileged citizens as about the importance of acknowledging the relationship between poverty and poor mental health. We have yet to find a way of putting the particular needs of people with disabling mental (and physical) conditions at the forefront of popular concern.

In the meantime, psychiatric hospital wards continue to close and in pursuance of a community care policy former 'patients' become ordinary 'citizens' and, as a result of ill-health or lack of work opportunities, 'claimants'. Some may not have handled money for a long time. Others may be quite unused to budgeting – the hospitals' effective systems of running patients' finances having removed control over drawing and spending money from the recipients.

From the very start of making a claim to the Department of Social Security, the person with mental health problems is at a disadvantage. It is not the responsibility of the local Department of Social·Security to check whether the claimant has applied for all the allowances that may be payable in their particular circumstances. The onus to make a claim and to make the right one lies fairly and squarely with the applicant. A claimant with intermittent episodes of poor mental health spoke about her experiences of the social security system at a recent MIND meeting.

You have to be articulate and determined to obtain your social security entitlements. Many people don't know how much money they should receive. They have to wait for weeks before any money arrives from the DHSS and they are frightened to query the amount in case they lose benefit while their circumstances are looked at again.[8]

At the same meeting the organizer of a busy London Citizens Advice Bureau commented,[9] 'Most people know next to nothing about the social security system. The little they do know has been picked up from the TV, relatives or friends ... They see the DHSS as remote, baffling and bureaucratic.'

In a survey[10] examining the living conditions of a group of patients discharged into the community, 91 of those interviewed were unemployed and relied on social security benefits as their main source of income after leaving hospital. However, nearly two-thirds said that no one had checked their benefit entitlement or whether they were clear how to claim prior to their discharge. Seventy-one people said they received no information at all, either on special grants for clothing or on single payments for furniture, and 43 said they had encountered a range of problems in claiming benefit after leaving hospital. Knowledge of the benefits that are available and advice on how to negotiate the complex Department of Social Security and housing benefit systems was clearly vital, but unforthcoming from the various agencies responsible for this group's rehabilitation.

This is by no means an isolated example of poor preparation for living in the community. Lack of information and difficulties experienced in pursuing a claim for benefit feature regularly in the enquiries received at MIND and other organizations involved in resettling people.

Not only is the process of claiming benefits difficult, claimants with mental health problems are often vulnerable to prejudice or hostility by those who administer the social security system and may even be excluded from their entitlements altogether. The following experience is not uncommon and highlights the conflicts that will continue to exist until there is a clearer understanding of the nature and effect of mental ill-health:

I got an appointment to see a member of staff at the DHSS who told me that I wasn't entitled to it [a furniture grant]. I knew my rights and told him them! He made comments such as, 'You don't look mentally ill to me', 'What is wrong with you?', and, 'When will you stop being ill?'. He was unhelpful and wouldn't say whether or not I was likely to get the money. In the end my social worker and my key worker at the hostel helped me to sort it out. I got the money but it was made so difficult for me to claim that many people would have been put off.[11]

What, then, is the current role of the mental health worker as adviser or advocate in the process of claiming welfare benefits? Social workers are commonly seen by their clients and the public alike as the people best placed to assist with welfare rights advice. Yet such a service is unlikely to be offered. Social workers receive little preparation or support for welfare benefits work and any assistance in this area is much more likely to be as a result of an individual social worker's own interest and enthusiasm than any formal training in this field.

All too often the best the social worker – or indeed any mental health worker – can do when financial problems are raised is to suggest the person goes to their local social security office to sort out the matter. Here, they will probably be faced with several hours' wait for attention, with no toilets and nowhere to purchase refreshments. The person behind the counter, underpaid and in a hurry, is likely to have no personal knowledge of the claimant and no understanding of how mental health problems manifest themselves. Neither is the social security officer likely to be familiar with the debilitating and often anti-social side-effects that accompany heavy medication and which will invariably slow down the interviewing process.

As the social security system finds itself increasingly under pressure from the growing numbers of people dependent upon it, social security staff struggle to cope in the face of cuts in their resources. The result, particularly in inner cities, is little short of a complete breakdown in the administration of the system, with literally thousands of claims outstanding and increased delays in payment. In such a situation, how can the claimant with mental health problems and the social security officer ever be in a position to match need with entitlement?

It is true that within agencies such as Citizens Advice Bureaux and local authorities, welfare rights practitioners exist to help bridge the gap between claimant and the Department of Social Security.

People with mental health problems have made several critical points here. First, the growth in numbers of the welfare rights worker with its own separate status and career structure is built, ironically, on the very backs of those people they purport to help. And although the help offered may yield more money in terms of unclaimed benefit, it is just as likely to be a confirmation of what the claimant already knows: that the level of benefits is simply too low to meet the cost of pursuing a life in the community like everyone else, however tightly you budget. No matter how diligent the welfare rights practitioner, he or she is as powerless as the claimant to manufacture the fundamental changes needed to improve the benefit structure and to overcome the stigma and prejudice that clings to those who engage with it. The remedies for those problems lie ultimately in the hands of the politicians and policy makers.

Secondly, 'help' in the form of advice and assistance in claiming benefit is overall patchy and inconsistent. Advice agencies such as Citizens Advice Bureaux often mirror the problems that the claimant encounters at the Department of Social Security – lengthy queues, long delays and a lack of awareness of poor mental health and the restrictions it imposes. In rural areas, welfare rights services may be limited or non-existent and may involve a difficult and expensive journey to reach them.

Thus, access to financial support for most people with mental health problems is a humiliating process which makes them feel inadequate and powerless; it involves surrendering their entitlement to other individuals who are in a stronger position to achieve results. Whereas in some cases this is appropriate, a more accountable, responsive and efficient social security system would allow many more people to deal themselves with the responsibility of establishing their right to their benefit. We have seen that financial support plays a key role in determining the success of a 'care in the community' strategy. We have also established that the way the current social security system operates cannot possibly provide the support needed for claimants with mental health problems to adopt an ordinary life in the community. A closer look at what is exactly on offer to meet their needs is equally discouraging.

Cash benefits for people termed mentally ill have largely been neglected as different governments have concentrated on introducing a variety of measures to remove people from the dole queue and make them 'productive' instead. The provision in the last 20 years of a rag-bag of disability allowances is aimed primarily at countering criticism of neglect of disabled claimants generally, rather than a serious attempt to embrace the differences, first between mental and physical conditions, and secondly within the diagnosis of mental illness itself.

The examples that follow serve to illustrate how poorly the benefit system caters for claimants with the same need for an adequate level of benefit, but possessing dissimilar disabilities.

The fairly recent availability of two tax-free and non-means-tested benefits – attendance allowance (for severely disabled people who need continual care and have done so for at least six months) and mobility allowance (for people who are unable or virtually unable to walk) – has undoubtedly benefited, in cash terms at least, some groups of disabled recipients within the community. A diagnosis of mental illness, however, gives you no access at all to mobility allowance and only in very limited circumstances to attendance allowance. The fact that this allowance is restricted to chronically sick and, in the main, physically disabled people who have difficulties in connection with their 'bodily functions', has in addition an adverse effect on informal carers. For unless the recipient of that care is eligible for attendance allowance, the provider will not qualify for the only benefit specifically designed for carers: invalid care allowance. Consequently, the majority of informal carers of people in mental distress receive no recognition at all within the state income support system. The extension of this allowance to married women in 1986, although welcome, also demonstrates that, although one form of discrimination has now been removed, action to remedy the unequal treatment of mental and physical conditions within social security legislation and practice is still outstanding.

The most recently introduced disability benefit, severe disablement allowance (SDA), illustrates just how difficult it is to fit poor mental health into convenient administrative categories. Like the extension to invalid care allowance, the introduction of SDA was hailed as an achievement in so far as it removed discrimination for male and female claimants (its predecessor required married women to demonstrate that their condition prevented them from carrying out normal household duties as well as showing incapacity for work). Yet such an optimistic view overlooks the fact that another form of discrimination has replaced the old. Those who apply for this new allowance must generally prove that they are both unable to work and have been assessed by a medical panel as 80 per cent disabled.

Introducing a disability test into the criteria for eligibility implies that the wide variety of behaviour that we term mental illness is capable of being reduced to a set of percentages. This is not an impossible task, providing the assessment system is properly designed and executed in order to elicit the degree of restriction on everyday activities that the mental condition imposes. However, the method of assessment currently used is quite inappropriate. It is rooted in the Industrial Injuries Scheme, which has for many years worked satisfactorily in awarding percentages to people who have suffered the loss of a limb or another physical disability. Thus, SDA claimants with physical conditions stand a much better chance of a fair and sensible assessment than those whose 'loss' is much less specific and more difficult to measure.

At the end of the day we are left with the question of why the government subjects claimants to such a stringent disability test at all, given that no state benefits can be seen to compensate for the extra costs and the other disadvantages mental ill-health exacts. The 'fringe benefits' of the social security system that are meant to protect the quality of life for vulnerable groups of people, such as free or concessionary travel and free prescriptions, are not automatically awarded to people with mental health problems. On the contrary, many find themselves excluded altogether, despite the fact that being able to afford to get out and being able to meet the cost of medication are vital if people are to be able to participate as ordinary citizens in the community.

In short, our system of welfare benefits is a poor tool for fashioning an effective 'care in the community' policy for people with mental health problems. In denying this group of claimants, who are unable to support themselves financially through work, a recognized place in society, the government remains wedded to the old stereotypes of the 'undeserving poor' and the necessity to control them. In that sense we have moved barely at all from the notions of poor relief that were established as far back as the Middle Ages.

Notes
1. Tony Novak, *Poverty and Social Security: Why the Poor are Always with Us*, Pluto Press 1984, p. 37.
2. Sheila Rowbotham, 'Travelling Public', *New Society*, 28 November 1986.
3. *The Health Divide*, Health Education Council 1987.
4. Eve Brook, *In Debt on Admission: A Study of the Financial Circumstances of Recently Admitted Patients*, University of Birmingham 1986.
5. *OPCS Report on Occupational Mortality; The Registrar General Decennial Supplement for Great Britain 1979–80 and 1982–83*, HMSO 1986.
6. *White Paper on Reform of Social Security: Programme for Action*, HMSO 1985.
7. Brian Abel-Smith and Peter Townsend, 'Challenging Government Assumptions', *Social Security: The Real Agenda. The Fabian Society's Response to the Government's Review of Social Security*, Fabian Society 1984, No. 498.
8. Jo Opie at MIND press conference 3 April 1986.
9. David Taylor at MIND press conference 3 April 1986.
10. Charlie Legg and Ada Kay, *Discharged to the Community. A Review of Housing and Support in London for People Leaving Psychiatric Care*, Good Practices in Mental Health 1986.
11. Jane Hartley at MIND press conference 17 September 1985.

11
Something to Do

CHRIS BUMSTEAD

Most people, including those of us with disabilities, feel that they need to be taxed in some way; they want their abilities and skills put to the test and use their sense of creativity. The obvious means used to be employment. But now that large numbers of the population cannot find jobs, a gap has appeared in people's lives and the problems this has been creating affect them economically, socially and psychologically. Job scarcity makes life for people with mental health problems doubly hard, not only because they are at the bottom of the pile in market terms, but also because for them, working means re-entering social life and becoming ordinary citizens again.

But let us go back a little and try to define 'work' – loosely put, it is *a meaningful use of time, energy and resources*. This implies that the worker gets something out of it, feels well-occupied and uses his or her skills and powers. Employment does not always fulfil these criteria. Admittedly it fills time, is usually rewarded in some way financially and will hopefully have some ultimate purpose. But jobs do not always call upon an individual's skills, initiative or creativity, nor do they always provide satisfaction or meaning – especially if the person is not directly involved in the creation of work and does not have the satisfaction of seeing the end product of his or her labours. This situation is particularly pertinent to the types of work available to those with mental health problems, through traditional work rehabilitation centres for example. The assumption seems to be that because someone has poor mental health he or she will be satisfied with repetitive menial jobs requiring little skill apart from concentration and perseverance.

Work in most psychiatric rehabilitation or sheltered work

139

centres usually means fairly simple production-line factory-style jobs such as packing, sorting or assembling. It does not require much initiative, problem-solving skills or design capabilities and due to its repetitive nature quickly becomes tedious and boring. Once you have learnt what motions to make to do the job correctly and easily, the interest wanes because there are no new decisions to make. Often learning the job is not even a creative process because the centre supervisors tell you exactly what to do and when to do it. So that the most potentially creative process – that of figuring out how to do the job – is denied to the worker from the start. And as if to add insult to injury, the reward that he or she receives at the end of a six-hour day, five days a week, is a pay packet of about £5. This may well be a cynical view of the sheltered work set-up and it has to be said that for some the daily structure, the activity, the chance to be with others, the sense of being busy and the fringe benefits of attending such a centre, make it worth their while. Nevertheless, I feel more imagination could be deployed to make the work experience in these centres more challenging and inspiring.

At this point it may be useful to look at what motivates people to work. The first thing that springs to mind is money. People go to work to get the money to feel financially secure. They want to be able to spend the money in a way that satisfies them in their time away from employment. Even if your idea of relaxation is watching television you still need money to pay the licence. A drink in the pub costs money, the cinema, a football match, visiting friends outside your neighbourhood costs money ... In order to be entertained, you have to pay. Those who live on state benefits know only too well; often they are not able to afford to participate in pleasures that most employed people take for granted.

However being employed does not automatically mean you have more money in your pocket to spend. This is particularly true if you have a disability or are emerging from a breakdown. The sort of salary or wage you are likely to receive is at the bottom end of the scale, especially if you have been out of work for a long time. In addition, unless you confine yourself to low-paid, part-time work, becoming employed normally means that your state benefits are discontinued and with it some of the other allowances such as free prescriptions, free dental treatment and reduction in help towards housing costs. It is therefore not always in one's best financial interests to be employed!

However, what we have been talking about is not really money as a motivation for work but remuneration for employment. Most people are willing to work for nothing – gardening, decorating, cooking, helping friends – but to be employed for nothing would be considered slave labour and thus unacceptable exploitation.

So let me start again; leaving aside the complex question of exchanging labour for money, what motivates people to work? Work provides a meaningful structure to the use of time; when you know you are using your skills and knowledge you feel that your efforts, time and energy are being used constructively; no matter how long you spend on a project, the ultimate satisfaction comes from seeing the job through all its stages and processes and finishing it successfully. There is nothing more disturbing than to spend your time purposelessly, to feel dissatisfied with not having anything to do; time drags, you become bored, lethargic, depressed and thoroughly pessimistic. The right kind of work can change all that. It can give you energy, interest, inspiration and a feeling of being alive. It can instil a sense of self-worth and respect. When you are doing something useful, you feel useful. In our society some jobs carry more status than others, but personal satisfaction carries a status all of its own. Having work to do grants you a position in society which demands the recognition of others, particularly if it is socially useful.

Another motivating factor for working is being with other people; working together means feeling part of a team, learning from others and sharing your own knowledge and responsibility. Working together usually involves some social contact which is taken beyond the working environment. All these factors add up to social involvement, acceptance and respect from others, as well as the feeling that you are needed and are playing a valued part in your community.

I have gone into the question of motivation for work at some length because the emerging principles should provide a base line for any work projects and schemes for people with mental health problems. If these motivational factors are ignored, there is a danger of repeating past patterns which lead to a stagnant and institutionalized environment.

But this is not meant to be a eulogy of work per se. Work can be very stressful. It requires concentration and stamina, is subject to various pressures such as expectations of customers and superiors, standards to be met, deadlines to be kept, contracts ... For someone who is prone to mental health problems, such added stress can be damaging and work could in effect be counter-productive. Monitoring what people are doing and assessing how much pressure they can take is therefore important; the work should be demanding but not excessively so. The work needs to be graded according to people's abilities, while at the same time allowing for progression and thus taking into account each person's potential. To minimize boredom there needs to be some in-built variety in the activity – there is nothing more soul destroying and numbing than having to do the same small task day-in day-out. The task of establishing a flexible median is one which demands insight, tact and a good relationship with all those involved.

The concept of work also implies some sort of structure – time, standards, authority, etc. Living one's life according to this externally imposed discipline is often very hard for people who suffer from mental ill-health as the latter can sometimes quite literally take over. The open employment market is not always flexible enough to respond to this sort of situation. There are of course sympathetic bosses who will make allowances, but they are by no means the norm. Consequently, any projects which provide work for vulnerable people need to be flexible and understanding enough to allow for the ups and downs of their workers and also to enable them to acclimatize gradually to a new lifestyle.

Let us now look at the sort of work alternatives there are currently available for people with mental health problems. First there is the open employment market. With rising unemployment and despite the efforts of Disablement Resettlement Officers (whose task it is to help disabled people find work), this service is unlikely to offer opportunities for the majority of ex-mental patients particularly as employers often discriminate against people who are or have been users of the mental health services.

Next come the Employment Rehabilitation Centres (ERCs) which provide assessment for employability and some skills training. However, because the ERCs are primarily geared towards getting their clients employed in the open market, this service is also limited.

In some areas there are community employment schemes which take on people who have either been unemployed for a long time or who have some disability (including mental ill-health). These schemes employ people for up to a year and pay a wage equivalent to state benefit levels while teaching people some basic trade skills. They claim to have a good record of clients subsequently securing employment, but this is of course again largely determined by current market vacancies. Another option is the factories run by Remploy. These factories aim to provide employment under industrial conditions as near to those in any other business. But here again the vacancies are few and there is some reluctance to take on people with a psychiatric history because of perceived potential management problems. So much for the open employment market!

Unfortunately statutory bodies such as the health authorities and local authorities are not at the moment providing a reasonable alternative. The former see their prime role as providing health services and the latter as supplying social support. Health authorities do provide day-care in the form of social and behavioural therapy but little attention is paid to work. The day-centres run by local authorities offer work possibilities but they tend to fall within the repetitive-numbing category as described before.

Although not leading directly to employment, another avenue to work is through further education and training which will provide the qualifications to compete on a more equal basis in the open market. There are many day and evening adult education classes available through which 'O' and 'A' levels as well as part-time degree courses can be taken without jeopardizing receipt of state benefits. There are also a variety of government training schemes specially designed for disabled people – for instance the Job Training Scheme (that replaces the Training Opportunities Programme) aims to teach new skills or develop existing ones and then provide work with an employer for a short period.

The obvious conclusion to be drawn from all this is that there are not enough suitable work facilities for the majority of people who have a mental health problem. It is therefore high time for the statutory bodies to re-examine their role vis-à-vis ex-patients. The forthcoming closure of large psychiatric hospitals around the country will release large amounts of money, which should be ploughed back into community services. Some of these should be work-orientated set-ups. They need not even involve a long-term financial burden on the health authorities – with the right approach and guidance, work ventures can fairly easily become self-supporting and self-generating, and even develop into small cooperatives.

Local voluntary organizations such as MIND have started to make some headway. A project such as Portugal Prints, which is a day-centre primarily set up as a small printing business and which actively encourages full participation of its members, shows what can be achieved. This initiative may of course have been possible because voluntary bodies are less hampered by the bureaucratic strictures of local and health authorities.

It seems that the key to success of any such work venture is to keep it small. This will prevent to some degree the danger of it becoming institutional, will help to promote a sense of cohesion and belonging amongst the workers, and allow them to take an active part in all the aspects, including planning and running, of the project. Another important factor is to set up a business that has a good chance of thriving; concentrating on something that is needed in the community where it is located. If it is a business it should be run, initially at least, by a business person, not a mental health professional. Ideally some skilled workers should be employed on a temporary basis at the start of the project so as to train and pass on their skill to the other workers. Naturally there may have to be some back-up from mental health professionals but this need not impinge upon the work environment.

The organization of day-care centres could also be shaken up. Clerical work, cleaning, looking after the garden, promoting and publicizing the centre, running a refreshments bar, are all jobs which could easily be done by users of the place. In addition, various projects could be set up to build or make things which would serve the members. In this way the day-centre is not just a place to receive a service, but it also becomes somewhere for people to make things for themselves and co-users.

An innovative way of providing employment for people with mental health problems, and one which has been successfully developed and implemented by Fountain House work project in New York, is the idea of transitional employment. The way this operates is that people work for a given period with a business to gain experience and then allow someone else to take their place. There is a proviso that if someone fails to attend for work a member of the staff of the centre which has arranged the placement has to fill in. This system works well at Fountain House because they have a large membership and sufficient members of staff. The initial problem of course is to find a firm that is prepared to employ people under this arrangement and to have enough people interested in doing the particular jobs on offer.

Yet another alternative is voluntary work. Although often maligned it is nevertheless very valuable and always highly appreciated. Thinking back to the motivations for working and forgetting about financial remuneration, voluntary work quite often fits the bill in terms of providing feelings of satisfaction and self-worth. There are many opportunities for doing voluntary work and the local Volunteer Bureau is the best place to find out about it.

For people who are in receipt of sickness benefit, invalidity benefit or severe disablement allowance, it is possible to earn up to £27 per week (1988 rates) in 'therapeutic earnings' without it affecting these benefits. This concession has been poorly publicized and it may require some searching to get all the details. There are now a number of volunteer workers who have taken advantage of the 'therapeutic earnings' ruling, which not only brings in some more money but probably also a feeling of self-worth.

Ideally work should reward people both financially and psychologically. Many of us have no choice in the matter and have to take whatever job is on offer just to keep abreast with the bills. But those of us who have a mental disability do not even expect to find a job! It is time for the authorities to come up with some viable long-term solutions. And maybe if these come in the shape of flexible work-scheme initiatives, there might be a surprise in store; instead of needing care in the community, the community might well start taking care of itself!

Part V
Power and Reaction

12

Hospitalized Psychiatry

HARRY REID

Until recently not much notice was taken of what happens to mentally distressed people. And this is reflected not just in the tiny amounts this country has been spending on their care, it is also demonstrated in the general lack of media interest and in the type of stories that have found their way into the tabloids when the subject of mental health is broached; it is either the supposed madness of a murderer or sex offender, or yet another episode of brutal treatment meted out to residents of a psychiatric hospital. Sensationalist reports such as these do not benefit anyone as they offer neither true investigation nor analysis. What they do is to reflect and reinforce a consensus based on fear: mentally distressed people are unpredictable and frightening and therefore best kept away from the rest of us; responsibility towards them has, for centuries, been fulfilled by mental hospitals which, though they may not always provide a first-class service, have the advantage of allowing us to forget about those frightening individuals.

This attitude is, to say the least, short-sighted, given that about 15 per cent of the population could expect to spend at least one spell in a psychiatric hospital during their lives, while yearly millions of people consult their GP with some form of emotional problem.

It is as if people have accepted a bargain; that in return for assuaging our unease and fear of mental distress we will put our fate in the hands of psychiatry. This means that we accept the psychiatric profession's claim that the experience of being mentally distressed can only be understood in terms of illness and that therefore as a branch of medicine specializing in these matters, psychiatry is the most appropriate agency to deal with

149

mental breakdown. Such a popular endorsement of psychiatry added to the powers provided by legislation, affords psychiatrists a great deal of authority as well as legitimizing their power.

Those practising psychiatry have the power to decide what is in people's best interests even if those individuals' own views on the matter differ considerably. This power is bolstered by a resistance to external criticisms of either their belief system or their methods. It goes like this: since mental distress is an illness, only those trained and with experience in psychiatry can know what they are talking about. Therefore criticism from 'outside' is invalid; 'outside', strangely enough, includes the people who have experience of mental distress. Appropriated by the experts, the mystification of mental health problems is completed by them withholding information from the users of their service.

Meanwhile the mental health services are generally regarded as being in a transitional state with the old institution-centred system being replaced by a more enlightened community-based approach. However, alarmingly few new facilities have emerged so far, and where they have, the medical hegemony continues, while the lack of any kind of control by those who use the services also persists. Same philosophy, same ideology on various smaller sites ... Does this reflect the spirit of community care? I thought it was supposed to enable people to take a greater degree of control over their lives and have a chance to live as ordinary people!

Hospital closure as part of the move to community care has attracted more journalists in recent years to look into the mental health services and to challenge the public's indifference. These articles and TV documentaries invariably paint a frightening picture of a humanitarian policy (community care) going disastrously wrong. And certainly, the figure of an ex-hospital resident being dumped onto the streets with nowhere to go has acted both as a focus for concern and as a media metaphor.

No matter how welcome this kind of media exposure has been in alerting slumbering public opinion, the reportage is generally based on a number of assumptions which must be challenged if we are to frame an adequate strategy to remedy the present situation. One of these assumptions is that there is an entity called society which has striven collectively to improve the plight of mentally distressed people. Another is that mental distress is an illness and that psychiatric intervention is the correct response. Based on these assumptions, a false conclusion is then drawn, namely that the present appalling implementation of community care is a temporary quirk which can be overcome simply with more resources, the nature of which is often left vague.

A more realistic view is that the mental health services have been at best an inadequate response to users' needs and at worst profoundly damaging. This is not overwhelmingly due to lack of finances but because the medical system is grounded in an ideology where 'doctor knows best'. And given the psychiatrist's additional powers this can at times take the shape of a severe case of authoritarianism which silences the users of the services.

The power of psychiatry can be explained by looking at what Foucault calls 'the history of the present',[1] for, as Marx observed, 'The tradition of all the dead generations weighs like a nightmare on the brain of the living.'[2] For people who are powerless as a result of mental distress, the traditions of past generations make the nightmare all the more trenchant.

A key to understanding psychiatry's rise is the fact that it has acted as a sponge, absorbing both criticism and alternative forms of practice where necessary. Examples include Tuke's moral treatment,[3] Freud's psychoanalysis, Maxwell Jones's therapeutic community movement[4] and most recently the language of community care. Thus psychiatry's eclecticism is also partly its power base.

But it is not possible to chisel out psychiatry's ascendancy in isolation from either the broad socioeconomic and political history of the times in which it emerged, expanded and consolidated its position. Nor is that power free from the narrower considerations of what is defined as mental illness.

Prior to the industrial revolution there was basically no specialist provision. People we now label as mentally ill were viewed essentially as part of an underclass, which also comprised criminals and other outcasts. They could be found in gaols and cellars or roaming as Tom O'Bedlams. Madness was considered to be a lack of reason which put people on the level of animals and which legitimized the brutal treatment they were receiving. Their subsequent physical separation into what were termed 'fitting receptacles' was not for their own good, but for the good of others. These 'fitting receptacles' were the asylums which emerged in the nineteenth century.

The development of asylums can be linked to the growth of a national market economy and with it an increasingly centralized state. As wage labour and work outside the home became more and more widespread, traditional coping and containment strategies within the family were being undermined. The state gradually took on this role and developed systems to police and control people's behaviour.

The system of poor law relief which had been developed during the Elizabethan era had become too expensive and was ideologically incompatible with the need for a supply of cheap labour. The 1834 Poor Law Amendment Act centralized the system, reducing the role of the parishes which previously administered relief. It also made the conditions for receipt of relief so undesirable, that only the poorest of the poor would apply. Indeed, the workhouse was grim and aimed to embue a work ethic and discourage malingering.

The mad posed a problem to the smooth running of the workhouse. Because they were disruptive they required a place of their own. Legislation was passed in the shape of the County Asylums Act of 1808 which allowed for public asylums to be paid for and built and later the 1845 Lunacy Acts made this compulsory.

Authority for the management of these asylums had to be vested somewhere. The basic function was containment and psychiatry manoeuvred its way into becoming the controlling group. Its claims were that madness had a physical cause and that as doctors they had the necessary technology for treatment. While their methods offered little proof to anyone interested in measuring their effectiveness, few people bothered to check. Then as now about a third of people spontaneously recover.

Psychiatry's rise, according to Castel,[5] falls into two eras. The 'golden age' which was characterized by the growth of a national network of asylums, takes us up to the middle of the nineteenth century; the second period brings us up to the present and includes the adoption of psychoanalysis and the so-called drugs revolution of the 1950s.

From the First World War onwards psychiatry became more and more a point of referral for both mildly and severely distressed people. Psychiatry's sphere of interest spread into families, communities, the army, industry, developing specialisms such as child psychiatry and forensic psychiatry, and setting the stage for an increasing psychiatrization of society.

Throughout, psychiatry's goal has been integration into medicine. The success of this policy has been manifested in the growth of psychiatric units in district general hospitals, a phenomenon which is now having a profound impact on the development of community care. Basically psychiatry borrowed medicine's clothes even though they did not fit too well. Western medicine is based on positivist science which requires, as far as possible, value-free objective observation. Psychiatrists deal with behaviour and in judging what is acceptable behaviour; they use the norms of a segment of society, thus setting themselves up as cultural arbitrators rather than as impartial scientists.

However, despite this and probably because people do not want to know, psychiatry's credibility has grown, especially with the development of a physical technology such as ECT, psychotropic drugs and psychosurgery. A reflection and consolidation of psychiatry's power are the alliances which it has forged during the course of the twentieth century with what are termed the 'psy-professions' such as social work and occupational therapy. However, these alliances which in their modern format find expression in the multidisciplinary team are by no means federations of equals with differing skills; they are invariably dominated by psychiatrists. Consultant psychiatrists in particular seem incapable of getting beyond understanding service provision in terms of what they perceive as the historical locus of their power!

Psychiatric authority presents a useful dimension for the state – that of control of deviance. Rather than suggesting some kind of conspiracy, I am merely pointing out a confluence of interests. Both the state and psychiatry consider that distress is caused by the individual's pathology, thus in this depoliticized version of reality, people are viewed as sufferers of illnesses rather than the victims of a harshly competitive society and an increasingly alienating way of living.

Ultimately, however, it is the state that holds the reins for it has political, financial and organizational control of the mental health services. Levels of power can best be envisaged as a system of concentric circles. In the case of the mental health services the outer all-embracing circle is the state, then comes the prevailing ideology of the time, followed by psychiatry. Whatever change is sought, one of these levels of power must be engaged.

For a truly revolutionary response to distress, however, there is first of all a need for an ideological shift in government coupled with a change in both the purpose of economic production and the people's relationship to it. The prevailing ideology of distress as a medical condition would have to be challenged, the social and political function of psychiatry either made redundant or renegotiated, and users of the mental health services treated as partners in their healing process.

But given that we are not on the brink of a revolutionary breakthrough, a transitional approach based on an understanding of the power of psychiatry might be more realistic. We must enter into a dialogue with psychiatry whatever we think of its function and methods, and persuade the profession that its true interests lie in non-institutional partnership – genuine community care.

But let us first look at the facilities emerging under the auspices of community care. A number of strands make up the totality of the service that is supposed to be replacing institutional psychiatric care. For many the mental hospital is being replaced by private residential care financed by social security payments. This trend was exposed in a 1986 report from the government's own Audit Commission.[6] Others, including a growing army of homeless ex-residents of hospitals, get no help at all, or at best the aid comes from informal carers.

The future for many of the elderly people at present in mental hospitals seems to lie with transfer to 'rump hospitals' in a rationalization process whereby one hospital becomes the designated one to remain open while others close; witness Banstead, Long Grove, West Park and Horton hospitals in Surrey. The plans are, having closed Banstead[7] by 'decanting' the majority of patients into Horton, to close the remaining hospitals by a process of transferring patients into two hospitals and ultimately into one. The other features on the road to community care are a hotchpotch of beleaguered social services, limited provision from the voluntary sector or a place in one of the growing number of private psychiatric hospitals or district general hospital units.

Precisely why psychiatric hospitals gradually started to close down is unclear. There does not appear to be one specific reason. The process of transferring people with mental health problems out of hospital more quickly started after the Second World War. Then there was the introduction in the mid-1950s of psychotropic drugs which control many symptoms of what is called mental illness. Another factor often mentioned is that the state could no longer afford to fund asylums, and that containment through drugs was cheaper. Certainly the climate of opinion was to support the move away from institutional care.

It is now clear that the liberal language of community care has been hijacked by the state for its own purposes as a cost-cutting exercise and that psychiatry views community care as just another opportunity to move to full integration with medicine. It will now deal only with the most 'interesting' people. The others with longer-term problems will be ignored and dumped or else come under the auspices of those psy-professionals such as social workers and nurses further down the hierarchical ladder. Thus community care as provided at the moment is a shift only in location; fundamental power relations are not changing. Indeed the spectre of compulsory community orders by which psychiatrists could enforce treatment on those living in the community is looming large and would further strengthen their position.

It would be foolish to say that there are no good psychiatrists, but good psychiatry is more often related to the empathy and respect such professionals show distressed people than with any technical expertise. However we must recognize that even they can wield enormous and indefensible power over other human beings. Full participation in our society is granted only to the powerful. In contrast, for those regarded as mentally ill, the marginalization process which began behind asylum walls is increasingly being replaced by invisibility in the community – a state of affairs so pernicious and deep-seated that only fundamental social and political change will alter it.

Those who wish to see improved aid for mentally distressed people prior to such radical change are left on the horns of a dilemma of whether to engage with psychiatry or try to set up alternative support and structures. However, the latter is only an option for the articulate and politicized survivors of the system. Psychiatry must be won over if the people most distressd and most damaged by the experience of breakdown are not to be left to the lions.

Notes

1. M. Foucault, *Madness and Civilisation – A History of Insanity in The Age of Reason*, Tavistock 1967.
2. Quoted in A. Scull, *Museums of Madness: The Social Organization of Insanity in Nineteenth Century England*, Allen Lane 1979.
3. See A. Digby, 'Moral Treatment at the Retreat 1796–1846' in W. F. Bynum, R. Porter and M. Shepherd (eds), *The Anatomy of Madness. Essays in the History of Psychiatry. Vol. 2; Institutions and Society*, Tavistock 1985. Also M. Donnelly, *Managing the Mind: A Study of Medical Psychology in Early Nineteenth Century Britain*, Tavistock 1983.
4. See R. D. Hinshelwood and N. Manning, *Therapeutic Communities: Reflections and Progress*, Routledge and Kegan Paul 1979.
5. For a concise outline of Castel's historiography see P. Miller, 'Critiques of Psychiatry and Critical Sociologies of Madness' in P. Miller and N. Rose (eds), *The Power of Psychiatry*, Polity Press 1986.
6. Audit Commission, *Making a Reality of Community Care*, HMSO 1987.

7. See H. Reid and A. Wiseman, *When the Talking has to Stop. Community Care in Crisis: the Case of Banstead Hospital*, MIND 1987.

13

Community Mental Health Centres – Rhetoric and Reality

LIZ SAYCE

'People's needs are the same, whether or not they have experienced breakdown.' This is a quote from a policy document about a community mental health resource, which I received in 1987 as part of a wide survey of British community mental health centres. It is a point that is made again and again in such documents, and one which, on the face of it, seems indisputable.

Or is it? The sentence actually could mean one of two things. It may be saying that everyone needs food and shelter; and moreover that needs for valued social roles and privacy are felt just as much by those with mental health problems (who thus should not be enclosed in large institutions) as by anyone else. Or it may be hinting at something different: not only that those people have no *less* needs than the rest of the population but also that they have no *more* needs. According to the latter version, having 'the same' needs means having an identical set,. the same in type and number.

This is unfortunately a perfect rationale for dismantling all special services for people suffering from mental health problems and ultimately all mental health provision: as long as restrictive and oppressive hospitals are closed, and the same opportunities offered for income maintenance and housing as to everyone else (or everyone else in social class 5, as is more to the point in practice) no more has to be done.

People with mental health problems do of course have the same needs as everyone else but they need more. The 'more' includes needs for positive action to counteract prejudice against them: for instance, projects which enhance access to housing, income or employment. Even more importantly, it includes

158

needs stemming from the mental health problems themselves
for a range of rehabilitative, therapeutic and treatment services.
This point is often ignored, because it is assumed that mental
illness arises only when people's universal human needs are not
met; therefore meeting their general needs, through ordinary
non-specialist services, should reverse the process and restore
psychological health.

There are two points of confusion here. First many mental
health problems do appear to stem from a collision between
people's needs and a hostile social environment; witness the
connection between depression and caring for young children,
as was established by Brown and Harris,[1] having no employment
outside the home. However, there is also a growing body of
evidence, embarrassing to a generation brought up on the ideas
of R. D. Laing, which suggests that a combination of environmental factors and biological predisposition can provoke the
more serious forms of mental illness.[2] The causes of a disorder
such as schizophrenia cannot be traced back solely to the social
level. Secondly, even if they could, it need not follow that intervention must occur at the same level (social, personal or biological) as that of the identified cause. Someone suffering from
dementia or schizophrenia, at least partly rooted in biology,
may benefit most from non-biological methods like behavioural
therapy or rehabilitation. Equally, once someone suffers from
depression, or a phobia, it is unlikely that they will be best
helped only by focusing on the social roots of the problem;
they also need skilled and well-planned help with its psychological impact. This is in no way to argue for retaining purely
medical models of treatment or indeed any methods that are
imposed without reference to users' views. It is rather to press
for a continuing exploration of alternative approaches and an
extension of those which actually prove helpful.

If these points are lost, so also is a coherent resistance to the
erosion of mental health services, which can then proceed un-
checked as a part of general welfare state cutbacks. This may
partly explain why the running down of large hospitals has
occurred at a faster pace than the creation of community

replacements – in the last ten years, 25,000 hospital beds have been lost, but only 9,000 new day places provided.[3]

Using ambiguous phrases like 'the same needs' or, for that matter, 'ordinary facilities', 'normalization' or 'community care', is dangerous in that ambiguities can be exploited and turned to the disadvantage of service users, potential users and professionals working on their behalf. This has happened most obviously with the notoriously nebulous term 'community care'. In the 1970s its meaning to policy makers, as expressed in the DHSS priority setting document *The Way Forward*,[4] was a growing public provision of day-hospitals, hostels, domiciliary services and so forth. By 1981, in an equivalent document *Care In Action*,[5] the emphasis was abundantly on the role of 'informal social networks'. 'Care in the community must increasingly mean care by the community', as one government spokesperson put it.[6] The emotional and financial burden placed on women in families (rather than the 'community') by the withdrawal of public services is well documented.[7] This shift in emphasis happened partly because a fake consensus on the value of 'community care' was established, grounded in the vagueness of the words. Until the mid-1980s, and in particular the Short Report's publicizing of shortfalls in community provision,[8] real disagreements about what needed to be done were rarely expressed, let alone resolved.

The most effective tool for resisting the evils of dehumanizing institutions on the one hand, and a style of 'community care' involving reduced services on the other, is the promotion of positive examples of community provision. This was a key part of the rationale for setting up a study of community mental health centres (CMHCs), still in progress, in 1987. CMHCs are of course not the only model of community service currently being developed. Other ideas include a variety of GP attachment schemes and sets of highly specialized community-based teams: for instance, Surrey's teams for rehabilitation, family interventions and alcohol abuse, or Hampstead's for people with chronic mental illness and for elderly dementia sufferers (the explicit idea being that other groups should continue to be served by general practice). The CMHC is, however, one model that is being adopted with some enthusiasm. Might this trend, or aspects within it, be one viable alternative both to the institution and to general service decline?

Community Mental Health Centres: The Context

Basing mental health services in the community is not a new venture. A decrease in the numbers of in-patients in the post-war period (from 3.4 per 1,000 population in 1954 to 1.5 per 1,000 in 1981) has been matched, if not at sufficient levels, by a steady increase in community provision. For example, numbers of new out-patients seen rose from 90,000 in 1949 to 196,000 in 1968.[9] Day-hospitals, numbering two in 1949, offered over 15,000 places by 1982.[10]

Of the variety of criticisms of community services that have been made during this period, from different vantage points, one of the most common has concerned a lack of clarity about aims and their translation into practice. Farndale, despite writing as an advocate of day-hospitals, found the movement behind their 'mushrooming' development hard to pin down because 'the term "day hospital" has a wide meaning'.[11] Local authority mental health plans in the late 1950s have been described by Martin as follows: 'For the most part, the statements of intent with regard to change in staffing, to ensuring training opportunities for existing staff, to providing residential and day care facilities, were couched in vague and general terms.'[12] This type of imprecision led Ramon to characterize the whole of community mental health development as piecemeal and 'pragmatic'.[13] Can the same accusations be levelled at the current 'mushrooming' of CMHCs?

When MIND put a parliamentary question concerning how many community mental health centres existed or were planned in Britain, they were met with the response, 'We have not so far sought either to define what minimum requirements would justify the term, nor therefore to obtain statistics on the number of centres within such a definition which are operating.'[14] This is not just a question of governmental evasion. Peck and Joyce have noted that every word in the phrase community mental health centre is ambiguous: it is unclear whether 'community' simply implies non-hospital based or whether it means a natural grouping with which people identify; whether or not a 'mental health' focus entails a departure from mental illness services in favour of prevention; and whether a 'centre' is a focal point for local people or simply a base for a team.[15] The phrase as a whole, admittedly, has a particular history, originating in the US and perhaps this can help to pin down its meaning.

CMHCs proliferated in the US, to a current figure of about 800 following the 1963 Community Mental Health Centres Act introduced by President Kennedy. Born in an era of high civil rights activity, they aimed to provide a free, local, accessible mental health service for all. Certain tensions, ideological and practical, have, however, characterized their development – a reflection, according to Levine, of social, economic, professional and organizational forces often working at cross purposes.[16] The centres themselves vary from large, well-equipped multi-professional units in the North East to small out-patients departments with the addition of one social worker in the South.[17] They have been accused in the 1970s and 1980s of a 'loss of perspective', often on the grounds that they have sacrificed effective help for people with chronic mental health problems to ill-defined social reform or counselling services for the 'worried well'. It is all very well, says Mollica, to remove obstacles to accessibility, such as class or race bias, but 'access to what'? The failure to pose this question and to find out whether services are actually effective has, in his view, led to a real threat of declining clinical standards.[18]

Conversely, the centres' radical potential in terms of community control and primary prevention has frequently been declared unrealized. Nassi claims that community control has been watered down to mean, at best, advisory participation;[19] and Good that the preventive 'consultation and education' component of the service is little more than a token, accounting for a mere 5.5 per cent of staff time.[20]

To the extent that these ambiguities and disagreements have brought discredit on the community mental health movement, they have made it vulnerable to cutbacks in federal funding, which have indeed occurred under the Reagan administration – the Omnibus Budget Reconciliation Act of 1981 mandated a 25 per cent reduction.

This picture hardly provides a clear and convincing model of what a CMHC is or should be. Even if it did, it is improbable that it could be transferred directly to Britain. The two countries have very different relationships between central and local government and different primary care delivery systems. Financial constraints on services are also distinct: for instance, the fact that only a narrow spectrum of medically orientated services are reimbursable under the public Medicare and Medicaid systems has had a very particular influence on the direction of US development, especially since reduced federal funding has increased the attractions for CMHCs of any alternative source of finance.[21]

If a CMHC 'package' seems not to have been transferred, one phenomenon that may have been is the ambiguity and danger of loss of perspective evident in the US experience. This point needs unravelling if vulnerability to cost cutting is not to be repeated in Britain.

Community Mental Health Centres in Britain

CMHCs first appeared on the British scene in the 1970s, established under the NHS (as in the London Borough of Lewisham's Mental Health Advice Centre), social services (Eastgate House in Sussex) or under joint management (Brindle House in Cheshire). By 1985 a list compiled by the King's Fund and updated by Good Practices in Mental Health identified 22 CMHCs and CMHTs (Community Mental Health Teams); although as this was not intended to be comprehensive, actual numbers were doubtless higher. My current survey suggests a further increase during the mid-1980s and a probability, based on the study of plans, of a sharper rise in the late 1980s and early 1990s. The survey is, however, still in progress, so the observations made here are necessarily preliminary.

It is also clear that exact numbers can only be established by imposing a single definition that may not coincide with others used in the field. I was as interested in finding out how many meanings the term had as in identifying the number of centres that fitted my own definition (which was 'a multi-professional, non-hospital-based centre, offering an easily accessible service including sessional therapy/support/treatment with individuals or groups'). A trawl for information from all UK health districts and boards, social services departments and health and social services boards rapidly revealed both a number of centres that fitted my description but did not call themselves CMHCs (for example, Lewisham's Mental Health Advice Centre); and, conversely, centres which *did* call themselves CMHCs but which offered something nearer a day-centre service – a structured weekly programme of groups and activities. The last phenomenon seemed more common.

CMHC has become something of a buzz word and many responses to my very factual questions almost suggested a sense that the particular authority thought it *should* have a CMHC. Some spoke of previously traditional day-centres being 'encouraged to adopt a community mental health centre approach to their work'; or of there being no specific plans, but 'broad proposals in some parts of the county' for CMHCs. Only a tiny minority gave a straightforward negative reply such as 'no such centres in this district'. All this may indicate a significant commitment to improvements in services, but it is extremely unclear what 'broad proposals' for CMHCs or a 'CMHC approach' actually involve.

An even smaller number of responses posed reasoned challenges to the term CMHC, in one case because the word 'centre' obfuscated the fact that community mental health developments are about concepts, not buildings, and in another because the word 'community', dropped from the particular team's title, was too vague to be meaningful. More precision of this kind is crucial if discussion about CMHCs and even planning proposals are not to be clouded in ambiguity.

If we cut through the linguistic uncertainty by looking only at those centres fitting my definition (over 100 operational or firmly planned centres identified to date), then certain common features do emerge. Policy documents, and aims cited in response to a questionnaire sent by me, suggest a number of typical values and practices. Policies tend to be framed with reference, on the one hand, to trends in community development advocated by key government publications (*Better Services for The Mentally Ill*,[22] the Short Report[23]); and, on the other, to certain philosophical ideas, notably as expressed in normalization theory and in influential documents such as MIND's *Common Concern*.[24] The keynotes are local, accessible, non-stigmatizing centres which provide a focus for an area's mental health service and encourage coordination between the NHS, social services and other relevant local agencies. Empowerment of service users is often stressed (for example, 'responsibility for effecting change lies mainly with the client'), sometimes with the corollary that this requires a lessening of the power of professionals.

How are these global ideas translated into practice? Most centres are a focus for local services, not in the sense that they are the point of entry for all new referrals (although this is envisaged, for instance, in Kent), but through combining a service that is 'comprehensive' (often excluding only those outside the 16–65 age range and those with primary problems of drug or alcohol abuse) with active cooperation with other agencies. For instance, the Hove Centre (in Sussex) collaborates with local branches of the National Schizophrenia Fellowship and The Association of Carers, who hold meetings on their premises; and the Tiverton Centre (in Devon) gives team members responsibility for liaison with particular key agencies or a number of GP surgeries. Such strategies, combined with a team made up of health and social services personnel, would appear to have great potential in terms of overcoming fragmentation between sectors.

Attempts to counteract stigma often involves use of an 'ordinary' house in a residential or shopping area and working methods that account for the social and personal, rather than only medical, aspects of mental health and disorder; hence, for instance, the common assessment procedure used by staff from all professions in the Lewisham Centre, London.

Maximum accessibility is often, although not always, attempted through a walk-in service or other method of self-referral. Either way, referrals in the vast majority of centres in fact come primarily from GPs. Research at the Lewisham Centre shows success in increasing the overall numbers seen by any psychiatric service for the catchment area.[25] The increase is accounted for primarily by people with emotional or situational disturbances who receive more substantial help at the centre than would be provided by their GP. Speeding up the process of obtaining help is also crucial. The Lewisham Centre, for instance, offers immediate assessment through its walk-in service and fixes a further session within a week if appropriate. Its crisis intervention team will see people within 24 hours or faster in an emergency. This contrasts with a route through multiple 'filters', for instance GP to psychiatrist to psychologist, underpinned by a typical wait of four to six weeks for an appointment with a consultant in adult psychiatry in the same health district. A few centres additionally have paid specific attention to attracting under-represented groups, such as black and ethnic minorities or women with young children; hence, for instance, the crèche at Gable House (South London).

The actual methods of work used are variable and have as yet been little evaluated. Users of Lewisham's walk-in service have, however, been shown to gain faster and greater improvements in social adjustment than were achieved by a control group referred to a local out-patients department.[26] Small-scale consumer studies at a couple of centres have demonstrated a high level of satisfaction: 76 per cent of the users who responded to a Gable House survey said they would return to the centre if they had future problems;[27] and 86 per cent of Coventry's Crisis Intervention Team respondents (not a random sample in that those with very brief involvement were excluded) said they found the counselling 'very helpful'.[28] The last group particularly valued the informal atmosphere and an approach that involved working with them to make changes in their lives.

This general picture suggests early evidence of real achievements in certain key and fairly commonly held aims. However, there are also divergences in CMHC practice, upon which hinge a number of central dilemmas. In some respects these dilemmas, like ambiguities in language, mirror problems encountered in the US.

The most crucial is the conflict between treatment and social reform. One strong motivating force in the CMHC movement has been a wish to reject a medicalized model of psychiatry in favour of a more holistic approach. Sometimes this goes along with a rejection of the whole idea of mental illness and an assumption, as described earlier, that people have the same needs whether they have suffered a breakdown or not. A substantial minority of centres so far surveyed have as their key aims such projects as promoting positive mental health in the community at large or enabling people to achieve their full potential. Support or treatment for those with long-term, serious mental illness appears either not at all or almost as an afterthought, as the last of a long list of aims. The Lewisham research showed that an accessible system drew people in from the virtually limitless pool of those with minor distress normally seen by general practice. Counselling the 'worried well', and certainly promoting community mental health, are literally tasks without end. Unless they are highly focused and undertaken as well as, and not instead of, work with long-term mentally ill people, this group's needs are likely to be squeezed out by the sheer pressure of work. This may be a particular danger given workers' possible temptation to pursue the greater therapeutic satisfaction inherent in work where change is more likely. It is also a danger when confusion about the causation of mental illness is prevalent: for those who, as described above, see all mental health problems as environmentally caused, and thus preventable, it makes sense to concentrate wholly on prevention. The evidence, however, is not on their side.

One solution is consciously to devote a section of the work to people with long-term mental illness. The Lewisham team, for instance, responded to the research evidence on the predominance of the 'worried well' amongst their users by establishing specific crisis intervention and rehabilitation teams, so as not to neglect those with diagnoses of psychoses. Other centres, like Gable House, Exmouth and South Tees, have set a priority on this group from the outset. Another solution is focused preventive work like the adult education class on relaxation run by the Tiverton team, their training for workers in Part III accommodation or the women's group and social club run from Gable House. Focused preventive work coexists in these teams with support for seriously mentally ill people: although resources can place constraints on the possible range (witness, for instance, the unpaid staff overtime that underpins much evening group work and educational work). Without careful attention to priorities, which must explicitly include people with serious mental illnesses (thus necessitating keeping the term or something very similar), CMHC work could degenerate into a very nebulous mission of altering a community's mental health or even its culture – an exact repeat of the 'loss of perspective' in the US, and one with all the same dangers of discredit for CMHCs, withdrawal of the psychiatric profession and ultimately sharp cuts in funding.

Paradoxically, as in the US, the general emphasis on reform is not matched by significant attempts to make services responsive to the views of service users or the wider community. Most centres surveyed have no formal input into policy for users or community representatives, although there are notable exceptions such as Nottingham's linked patients' councils and team-based user groups, or Manchester's Powell Street community planning group, whose representatives have real influence in centre management, holding key chair and secretarial positions in training and evaluating sub-groups. Quite a few centres state that they have no specific links with the local 'community' at all. These points throw some question on the two common aims of 'empowering users' and 'creating social networks and a sense of belonging through community links'. They may also lend support to the action of the team mentioned earlier who dropped the excessively vague word 'community' from their title, although removing the word does not in itself resolve the question of what roles local groups and service users can play in the centres.

If these overarching and ideological dilemmas are critical, so too are the more pragmatic concerns of organizational functioning. I shall concentrate on one especially thorny issue: difficulties in multi-professional teams in terms of locating power and responsibility. Contradictory policies on subjects like access to files may filter down different professional management lines and areas of responsibility within teams may be left uncertain in the complex process of interdisciplinary skills sharing. A variety of strategies have been developed by CMHCs to tackle these problems: management or advisory groups to enhance collaboration between line managers in different professions; permanent psychiatrist/director posts; permanent or rotating coordinator posts from any profession; or democratic, consensus models. None of these is without potential pitfalls. Coordinators may have 'responsibility without authority', in the words of one team. Psychiatrist/directors may lessen the potential of skills sharing, as was apparent in one team when the post ceased, at which point various dilemmas emerged concerning the relative weights to be given to medical or other models of care. Consensus models can involve an element of pseudo-democracy: 'you don't hear doctors saying "I really must get a non-medical opinion on this" ', as one team member told me in a recent local *Good Practices in Mental Health* study.[29]

These issues are further complicated by the numerous possible locations of clinical responsibility, as revealed by responses to my questionnaire: it may rest with the team's consultant psychiatrist, with the user's GP or with all qualified professionals in the team. Its location may vary within a single team: one team stated that if a consultant made a referral to the team he or she retained responsibility; another that referrals could be made specifically *to* the team's consultant, in which case he/she rather than the whole team became responsible. These variations mirror the extreme ambiguity that surrounds the question of where legal responsibility for cases should lie, or even where it does lie as evident in the radically different views held nationally by relevant professional bodies.

There is a common belief amongst consultants that they could be held legally responsible if a patient caused harm to himself or others, even if a completely different professional had dealt with the case. According to the Royal College of Psychiatrists, this is right and proper: consultants, by virtue of their training and the fact that the medical role is the 'prime mover for the whole process of treatment and care', must take on the responsibilities of clinical leadership in multidisciplinary teams.[30] According to the British Association of Social Workers, by contrast, or the Psychologists' Protection Society, psychiatrists should never be held responsible for the judgements of a psychologist or social worker, who are after all independent professionals, not paramedics. Consultants, according to this viewpoint, should not conduct their caseloads as though sitting in a coroner's court. Nor should they use spurious arguments about legal responsibility as a cover for protecting their privileged status.

A key problem here is the relative lack of case law, as yet, in the sphere of multidisciplinary community psychiatry. What is clear is that it is a misconception, and a commonly held one, that consultants can be held responsible for the negligence of other professionals; 'a multidisciplinary team has no "commander" in this sense', as the Nodder Report puts it.[31] However, the actual situation, that each professional is responsible within their own area of competence, begs as many questions as it resolves. Where exactly is the boundary between a psychologist's, as opposed to a doctor's or social worker's, area of competence? Until more precedents are established uncertainty is likely to breed caution amongst professionals. Psychiatrists, for instance, may feel loath to rely on the Medical Defence Union's view (correct, although in this specific field still largely untested in court) that doctors can only be responsible for another professional's work if directly supervising them.

If legal uncertainties could be resolved, one (although clearly only one) obstacle to effective skills sharing in multidisciplinary teams would be removed. This might also go some way to overcoming the confusion which is currently, and not surprisingly, felt by many service users concerning who is accountable in relation to them.

There is no single blueprint for a successful management structure. It is clear that many teams are grappling with the dilemmas, trying for instance to maintain effective team work by being utterly clear about the task and by counteracting informal deference to single professions. It is an area of complexity, however, which will continue to require 'grappling with' in the future.

Conclusion

CMHCs are expanding rapidly in Britain. The term is, however, used to apply to a number of different models; and some of the central elements of the CMHC enterprise, for example counteracting the stigma associated with mental illness, are shared with other forms of service, such as teams that are not centre-based. The growth of CMHCs does not therefore constitute a self-contained 'movement'. Even so, CMHCs share certain key aims, such as providing a focal point for local mental health services and offering a swift, local and accessible service. They appear to be meeting these aims with some success. As one innovative form of community provision, they therefore hold great potential.

For this potential to be realized, a number of critical issues need clarification: the meaning or at least the clearly enumerated *meanings* of the term CMHC; the balance being attempted and achieved between prevention, social reform and treatment; the methods by which CMHCs can belong to the 'community', for instance, by instigating mechanisms for community and user participation in decision-making; and certain dilemmas concerning organizational structure and the location of clinical responsibility. There is no need for a quest for a single blueprint;

different localities, for example rural and urban areas, will require different forms of service. But without increased clarity at centre level there is a danger of loss of perspective both locally and in the more general national debate.

Research methods pioneered at Lewisham's Mental Health Advice Centre and computerized case registers developed at the 608 Centre in Waltham Forest, London are invaluable tools in beginning to assess CMHCs' achievements. There is, however, still a paucity of evaluative research – a gap that needs urgently to be filled if current developments are to be based on fact rather than rhetoric. Increased communication between centres in different parts of the country is also necessary. Few centres have substantial links with others of their kind. Difficulties in finding time for mutual visits are common, despite a strong commitment to learning from others' experiences. Policymakers need to ensure that monitoring and coordination are given the priority that they deserve.

Piecemeal developments which are not based on sufficient data or clear analysis have purportedly led to the following syndrome in US mental health developments: 'Fashions and fads in treatment, based on inadequate data, somehow attain cultural status as validated wisdom, and these ideas affect public policy.'[32]

British CMHCs have neither reached this stage, nor have they achieved a clear model or models from which to argue for the necessary direction of development. Two possible routes lie before them: drifting into a lack of perspective, concealed behind a fashionable name, with an ultimate danger of loss of credibility with the next change of fashion; or sharpening their focus and basing their growth on evidence of their very real potential. The opportunity to take the latter path is there now; it might not be in ten years' time.

Notes

1. G. W. Brown and T. Harris, *Social Origins of Depression*, Tavistock 1978.
2. I. I. Gottesman and J. Shields, *Schizophrenia, The Epigenetic Puzzle*, Cambridge University Press 1982.

3. Audit Commission, *Making a Reality of Community Care*, HMSO 1986.
4. DHSS, *The Way Forward*, HMSO 1977.
5. DHSS, *Care in Action*, HMSO 1981.
6. DHSS, *Growing Older*, HMSO 1981.
7. Equal Opportunities Commission, *Who Cares for the Carers?*, Equal Opportunities Commission 1982. J. Finch 'Community Care: Developing Non-Sexist Alternatives', *Critical Social Policy*, 9, 1984.
8. Social Services Committee, *Community Care with Special Reference to Adult Mentally Ill and Mentally Handicapped People*, HMSO 1985.
9. F. M. Martin, *Between the Acts, Community Mental Health Services 1959–1983*, Nuffield Provincial Hospitals Trust 1984.
10. Social Services Committee, *Community Care*, para 90.
11. J. Farndale, *The Day Hospital Movement in Great Britain*, Pergamon Press 1961.
12. Martin, *Between the Acts*.
13. S. Ramon, 'The Logic of Pragmatism in Mental Health Policy', *Critical Social Policy*, Vol. 2, No. 2, 1982.
14. *House of Commons Parliamentary Debates, Weekly Hansard*, 2 December Col. 143–4, HMSO 1985.
15. E. Peck and L. Joyce, 'Community Mental Health Centres – A View of the Landscape' in T. McAusland (ed.), *Planning and Monitoring Community Mental Health Centres*, King's Fund 1985.
16. M. Levine, *The History and Politics of Community Mental Health*, Oxford University Press 1981.
17. K. Jones, 'Lessons from Italy, the USA and York' in McAusland (ed.), *Planning and Monitoring Community Mental Health Centres*.
18. R. F. Mollica, 'From Asylum to Community. The Threatened Disintegration of Public Psychiatry', *The New England Journal of Medicine*, Vol. 308, No. 7, 1983.
19. A. J. Nassi, 'Community Control or Control of the Community? The Case of the Community Mental Health Center', *Journal of Community Psychology*, Vol. 6, 1978.
20. P. R. Good, 'Brief Therapy in the Age of Reagapeutics', *American Journal of Orthopsychiatry*, Vol. 57 (1), 1987.
21. R. L. Okin, 'How Community Mental Health Centres are Coping', *Hospital And Community Psychiatry*, Vol. 35, No. 11, 1984.
22. DHSS, *Better Services For The Mentally Ill*, HMSO 1975.
23. Social Services Committee, *Community Care*.
24. MIND, *Common Concern*, MIND 1983.
25. A. P. Boardman, N. Bouras and J. Cundy, *The Mental Health Advice Centre In Lewisham. Service Usage: Trends from 1978 to 1984*, NUPRD 1987.

26. Ibid.
27. Gable House Team, 'Results Of The Gable House Clients' Survey', unpublished 1987.
28. A. Davis, S. Newton and D. Smith, 'Coventry Crisis Intervention Team: The Consumer's View', *Social Services Research*, Vol. 14, No. 1, University of Birmingham 1985.
29. L. Sayce, *Good Practices in Mental Health, Lewisham And North Southwark*, NUPRD 1987.
30. K. Rawnsley, 'The Future of the Consultant in Psychiatry', *Bulletin of the Royal College of Psychiatrists*, July 1984.
31. DHSS, *Organizational and Management Problems of Mental Illness Hospitals. Report of a Working Party*, DHSS 1980.
32. Levine, *The History and Politics of Community Mental Health*.

14

Changing Our Professional Ways

ANDREW MILROY AND RICK HENNELLY

Power and powerlessness are central experiences for everyone involved in the provision or use of mental health services. For those of us with the responsibility to provide services, the exercise of professional discretion and judgement involves the use of power over fellow citizens who turn to us for help. People using mental health services lose, forfeit or actively seek to dispose of power and control over their own lives. The character of modern professional health and social services is such that loss of power is inevitably encouraged. Our society has generated strong images of omni-competent professionals who soothe, cure and remove the hurt, pain and problems of living. These images are deeply ingrained in our culture; users of professional services are as eager in their expectation of a painless solution, as we are willing to supply it. The 'oppressed' have 'internalized the image of the oppressor and adopted his guidelines (and) are fearful of freedom'.[1] Citizens and professionals participate in an act of subjugation and domination, performed in every encounter. Professional power and professional solutions are acknowledged and strengthened at the expense of the personal competence and the ordinary solutions of the citizen.

All too often this power is exercised in ways which mirror the social, political and economic order of our society. The social and economic disadvantages which both spring from and cause 'mental breakdown' are perpetuated by the exercise of reformist professional power, shaping problems to fit the available solutions and rooting both at the level of individual action. Social, political and economic contexts are removed and the problems of each person are shaped by the remedies available. Problems are concerns on which to impose new 'helping technologies' or 'social engineering'.[2] People, usually from a different social class and living in a different area to the professionals, are clients to be 'worked on'.

The growth of new 'techniques' in services invariably emphasizes the indispensability of professional solutions. Professional mental health services are taken into ever-increasing areas of ordinary human experience. Disease, individual pathology, and dysfunction, promote the interests of the expert. In this process, the correctness of the assumptions of each profession is confirmed by the growing numbers of 'consumers', most of whom have been well-'educated' to accept and even desire the ministrations of the professional service. The growth of the widespread belief in professional solutions ensures that human wants become transformed into professionally defined needs. The ultimate in this process is that mental health problems are any problems capable of being solved by professional effort. Professional technology is seen as the solution and human despair is not to be acknowledged unless professional technology can respond to it.

The paradox of this subtle (although at times not so subtle) transfer of power from citizen to professional, goes on unremarked. The acquisition and expansion of professional power and status infects the aspirations of all professions. The 'achievements' of psychiatry, accruing, as it has been, disproportionate status in mental health services, is emulated by psychology, social work, nursing and others. And as professions they struggle to gain advantage over each other. Each is always assured at the very least, of supremacy over the citizens who become passive consumers of their professional services.

Things that Must Change

As our mental health services are reorganized to try to achieve community integration, it is time for us to examine how we can change the character and use of our professional power. The imperatives for such changes are the rights and dignity of each of us as ordinary citizens and the demands of effectiveness. If our professional power limits or prevents people who experience mental distress, from gaining control over their own lives, as we believe it does, it challenges our legitimacy. How can we reshape our practice? How can we achieve a state of 'working with' rather than 'working on' people?

The following ideas arise out of the work of the North Derbyshire Mental Health Services Project based at the Tontine Road Centre in the middle of Chesterfield. They also reflect the experience of many colleagues who work in the district, but most importantly, they mirror the thoughts and achievements of the men and women who have come to use the mental health services in North Derbyshire. Their endeavour shapes our practice and validates our actions.

Accountability

Developing a finely tuned sense of accountability is a prerequisite for 'working with' people. This sense of accountability must be directed towards the men and women who use our services, the communities in which people live, the social and political institutions of our society and our employers. Accountability involves a commitment to respond to the questions, challenges and directives of the people we are concerned to support. It is rooted in a firm belief that professional activity is a tool of the ordinary citizen and has no monopoly on truth and wisdom.

The following illustrates what we mean by accountability. The Tontine Road Centre, which provides a base for the North Derbyshire Mental Health Services Project, is used by over 33 community groups and services. The organization and operation of the centre is focused through a Management Committee made up of representatives of all the groups using the facility.

The social support groups we have developed which provide a focus for the work of the project, are all formally constituted self-regulating independent community groups. Project workers and other colleagues have and accept specific responsibilities to provide material advice and support. The constitutions of these groups establish a form of 'Service Charter' setting out the rights and duties of those providing the service as well as those using it. The extension of the use of some kind of charter for other aspects of our services needs further consideration. A charter challenges the ultimate power of professionalism – the power to make and alter unwritten rules, manipulate procedures, and maintain control.

There are 'resource exchange networks' referred to currently as Local Planning Groups, in each of the four areas making up North Derbyshire. These groups draw together all those people in the area who have an interest in or a contribution to make to community mental health services. All the Local Planning Groups are open ended, having no fixed constituency other than that defined by the mailing list. This aims to maximize the involvement of ordinary community groups.

Specific projects have been initiated by ordinary citizens making demands on the service. The local branch of the National Schizophrenia Fellowship, Creswell Open Door Club, West Derbyshire Mental Health Federation, Listening Ear (a support group for bereaved parents), Contact (the main social support group in Chesterfield) and others, are all examples of demand-led activity supported by mental health workers in the district. Allowing ordinary citizens to set the 'agenda' and direct the development of professional activity ensures that genuine alliances and partnerships can emerge.

Accountability to individuals is equally important. Harry was 53 when we first met him. He was living in a long-stay hospital some 18 months after his transfer on licence, from a secure hospital. Harry had spent much of the past 20 years in hospital. In recent times, attempts to get him out had failed as he actively rejected hostels, half-way homes and day-centres. A year after leaving hospital he now lives on his own. When he first moved into his house, a small team of workers spent some time living with him. The level of support was gradually reduced until after 11 months he was receiving no more support than is routinely available to any other person using the project. At no time during the past two years has he become formally involved in any of the sheltered occupational or leisure activities. He has chosen to remain on the periphery of the system, supported in a way he has found satisfactory.

Eric approached one of the social support groups. He was unemployed and wanted to do some voluntary work. It was clear that he had many difficulties, in particular, a serious drinking problem. Fortunately, the culture of the group, which builds its relationships around skills and abilities, allowed him to join on his terms. Gradually, during the past two years he has been able to tackle his own difficulties without the need to disable him by turning him into a 'client' or 'patient', a decision he would have strenuously resisted.

Accountability to individuals is expressed by the 'Ordinary Life Strategy' adopted by Derbyshire County Council.[3] This provides funding and a policy framework which allows us to build the kind of support people prefer and which reflects dignity and respect for individuals. The policy makes it possible to develop services which reflect the common values we all share. Finance is available to provide intensive support so that individuals can remain in their own homes with appropriate assistance. The 'Ordinary Life Strategy' moves us towards models of self-regulated care and support, which emphasize the importance of ordinary relationships and social experiences. This is backed by flexible and responsive professional help which begins to provide the required continuity of care and assistance.

Although there are still problems about funding long-term support, a service is now emerging which acknowledges the traditional criticism of mental health services, that they 'define their responsibility for people with severe mental disabilities narrowly'. Services all too often become '... concerned with "treatment" in the form of verbal therapies and medications for co-operative people ...' and neglecting the need to build community support for people who fail to 'get better'.[4] Funding effective and appropriate ways of supporting seriously disabled people and the families concerned with them, is a crucial part of 'working with' people.

Building Alliances – Participation and Partnership

'Working with' people requires us to identify with the cultural, social and economic experiences of any area. We must be sensitive to the real priorities for change. It is all too easy to misdirect energy and financial resources into efforts aimed at ameliorating problems which have their roots in the social and economic difficulties of a community. There seems little point to call for increased mental health services to deal with the rising incidence of human distress which we know to be directly related to growing unemployment, poor housing and low wages for those in work. Neither can we afford to neglect the influence of faltering community services – social, educational and environmental – which squeeze the quality of life for the majority of people with whom we are concerned.

We must play an active part in the ordinary concerns of communities. In one instance this meant taking part in the struggle to secure local community facilities. Elsewhere it was helping to set up a tenants' association, or developing close links with local centres for unemployed people. Most of the people who we will be principally concerned with face a lifetime of unemployment and many of those face mental health problems.

Our involvement with and support of the local branch of the National Schizophrenia Fellowship, MIND, Chesterfield Churches' Association for Social Work, North Derbyshire Council on Alcoholism, Samaritans, amongst others, provides a valuable contact with community groups which express a particular concern with our work. At times, the views and objectives of these groups will conflict with our own. It is important though that we acknowledge their independence. They are not adjuncts to our professional service but legitimate expressions of the concerns of ordinary citizens.

Supporting the participation of users of mental health services and voluntary sector groups (MIND, National Schizophrenia Fellowhip, etc.), in the planning, organization and delivery of these services, is crucial. Building a service together is about sharing problems and sharing power. The emphasis is on active participation by individuals in providing a framework which allows solutions to be found for their difficulties. The emphasis is also on mutuality, in the recognition that cooperation is a desirable state of affairs. No one has all the answers and everyone has problems of some description. Control is an issue and controlling relationships and distinctions such as doctor/patient, therapist/patient, professional/client are avoided, since these involve the abandonment of an individual's sense of confidence and purpose.

However, the use of our professional power to establish this framework of experiences within which people can gain access to power for themselves, cannot and should not deny the power which remains with us. It is not an exercise in the denial of reality. We remain doctors, social workers, nurses, psychologists. What changes is not this reality but how the reality is expressed. We cannot speak for people and we must stop trying. Our task is to give credible platforms to individuals and groups so that they can articulate their own demands. Advocating and providing clear tangible evidence of the value of services controlled and organized by the men and women who use them is essential. Our expertise must be committed to acknowledging the validity of user-controlled services. Submitting ourselves to act on the directions of the people we support is our declaration of their competence and legitimacy. Chamberlin (1978) outlined a model for a good alternative service for 'ex-patients'. In this model 'help is provided by the clients of the service to one another and may also be provided by others selected by the clients. The ability to give help is seen as a human attribute and not as something acquired by education or professional degree.'[5]

We can build alliances with groups of people who use services. Such groups often come together spontaneously when people wish to rid themselves of their isolation and explore mutual problems with others. We can help such groups to link up with one another, help them to have a voice by supporting their access to facilities which aid their development as a group, for example let them use our phones, our meeting rooms, our typewriters, our photocopiers. Better still, help them get their own.

Involvement with trade unions, churches, business associations, clubs, schools, youth groups and the like, becomes a routine part of the process. Participation by workers in the local trade union council and involvement in a 'Concern Network' enables us to build alliances and develop a clearer perception of the priorities for ordinary people. Through this process, we can also identify the natural strengths and resources of our communities, enabling us to link people into ordinary sources of support.

Alliances must also be developed between all those professional workers who make up a community mental health service. For us that means sharing in the problems colleagues face. The North Derbyshire Mental Health Service Project operates as an open access service enabling community psychiatric nurses, general practitioners and others to use facilities directly. We also provide funds for groups run by colleagues as well as contributing to joint projects. The minibus is available for anyone to use, and video equipment can be borrowed. These things help us to build mutual trust and confidence as well as to pool resources.

Building on Skills and Abilities

We can change our relationship towards each person who turns to us or our service. Such a change should emphasize getting to know each person as a whole, acknowledging skills and abilities as well as problems of living. Building on shared social experiences gives us access to relationships grounded in the present rather than in the past, which in turn allows us to emphasize and strengthen personal competence. This changed relationship will involve eliminating unnecessary 'professional distance', whilst still acknowledging the reason for our relationship. Time and interest in the difficulties people face in their lives will become critical components of effective strategies to help and assist people. We will be working 'with' rather than working 'on' people. Within this social process, treatment in all its forms, is relegated as a tool of the task of supporting people, rather than the task itself.

Political Action

Acting politically is essential. We can use our position to high-light the essential need for political change and we can support people as they struggle to face change. For us this has meant getting involved with a group of homeless women to help them articulate their demands for change in the quality of services they receive.

Behind medical 'explanations' and the widespread use of prescribed drugs in GP surgeries or psychiatrists' clinics lie a wealth of problems located in social, economic and political circumstances. We need to respond to these problems by arguing for support to be provided in locations chosen by individuals, at the level they request. 'Medical judgements' are often shallow and short-sighted. It may be important to go beyond them and tackle entrenched difficulties in relationships or social circumstances. When medical judgements are made, it is usually helpful for us to be persistent in enquiring why they were made and whether information is properly shared about the consequences of such judgements; for example, information about the side-effects of major tranquillizers or the short-life effects of minor tranquillizers. In more extreme circumstances, the proposed use of ECT must always be challenged. Its value is not just a matter of 'scientific debate' but is of concern to us all as a procedure of dubious origin and moral legitimacy.

We can bring issues to trade union meetings, for example the 'conscience clause' in contracts for nurses who are unhappy about being forced to participate in psychiatric procedures with which they disagree.

We can try to extend the democratic control of planning pro-cedures which have traditionally been the preserve of distant 'professional planners'. At the same time, we can make links with sympathetic individuals in policy-making bodies who are prepared to take up the issues. In particular, elected councillors on social services and health district committees should be sought out.

We can argue for our department, employer, team, unit and

the like, to have a value base or set of principles for service delivery. Such statements can be used as levers to challenge and change unhelpful and undemocratic practices and attitudes, or policies which take no account of the individuals who will be most affected by their implementation.

Once again the challenge is to effect change *with* not *to* people who use mental health services. The struggle to transform the social services or health service is the same struggle to transform the lives of those who are affected by the operation of these institutions and who may spend a great deal of time in contact with them. To give a sense of value to those people who experience profound disturbance of thought, feeling or behaviour, it is important to create a climate in which those of us who are employed to provide a service to such individuals, also feel valued. This means giving a voice to people who are affected by mental health services, in the creation of these services. Change requires participation.

Conspiracy of Confidentiality

Activities which exclude people who use services and which seek to create 'classes' within our services must be attacked. This might mean opening up hitherto 'confidential' files. It might mean questioning whether discussion about people who use the services is necessary in their absence. It might mean inviting them to social events, conferences, meetings from which they have traditionally been excluded. This is about recognizing the variety of strengths that people can demonstrate even when they have disabling internal experiences, and about recognizing their essential 'humaneness'. It means altering the balance of forces within traditionally 'closed' networks of professionals and requiring dialogue with, rather than about, individuals.

Confidentiality issues must be explored since several contradictions are thrown up in community settings. For instance, individuals have a right for information about them to be withheld from others if they so wish, but the creation of supportive community networks often implies that knowledge about people is shared.

Changing our Language

Our way of speaking and the development of jargon bolsters professional power, denying ordinary citizens access to the ideas and issues we seek to deal with. Jargon often obscures and mystifies the obvious and reduces the sense of competence people feel. We have been present in meetings involving ordinary citizens and members of community groups, where the style of language and the use of jargon effectively eliminated the useful participation of community members in what was being discussed. The contributions of ordinary people were often disconnected from what was being discussed by the professionals. The professionals through this experience simply confirmed their prejudices that the extent to which ordinary people could usefully contribute was very limited. Yet most of the subjects were simple and ordinary, concerning housing, GP care, jobs and recreation. We must attempt to discuss ordinary things in ordinary ways, if we are to involve ordinary people. Building alliances implies a balance of power and a sharing of information. It also implies acknowledging that we as professional mental health workers do not have all the answers but are prepared to share our skills and energies to help people discover the solutions they find most appropriate to their problems and the problems of their communities.

We can use a language which omits references to discriminatory attitudes and values. We can also try to describe experiences without the use of convenient but unhelpful medical labels. Even were we to accept the concept of 'mental illness', it would only cover a minority of the mental health problems which we all experience from time to time. Terms like 'chronic schizophrenic' and 'personality disordered' do not mean a great deal and often obscure the nature of real human needs as well as consigning individuals to 'cannot be helped' categories. Some of the terminology of psychiatry is as offensive as racist or sexist language is – it denies the real value of the person about whom it is used. Unhelpful phrases can often be avoided by referring to the description of experiences which people offer us to express their distress and by paying attention to their wishes and aspirations.

Information and Education

We must spread information about good practices in mental health and help people to feel in touch with others for support or simply to find out what is going on elsewhere. We can also try to establish wider discussion by encouraging concerned groups to get together on occasions, for example relatives' groups, church groups.

Through this we can seek to rebuild a sense of citizen competence in matters concerning the difficulties we can all experience in our thinking, feeling and behaviour. We can help to reclaim a range of ordinary human experiences from the realm of the incomprehensible and the unspeakable.

Changing Where We Work

Working with people means using the ordinary facilities available to everyone. Securing special facilities entrenches deviant images and often reflects our concern not for the needs of the community but rather our need for professional power and status. It is also more comfortable and less threatening for us. The development of special facilities also reduces the extent to which we will look to exploit the ordinary facilities and organizations of our communities which may more often be more appropriate.

The North Derbyshire Mental Health Services Project works from a multi-purpose centre in the middle of Chesterfield. The fact that the project is responsible for the building develops an 'institutional inertia' which inhibits our work with the community. However, this is offset to some extent by the way the centre is managed, as we explained before, and the fact that with the exception of two small offices providing insufficient room for all the team at once, all space in the centre is available to all groups and individuals and must be booked in advance by everyone, staff included.

For the out-reach programme, project staff work in outlying districts of North Derbyshire. The physical facilities used so far involve community and adult education centres, pubs, church halls, cafés, leisure centres, people's homes, clubs and the like. Our experience suggests that we should avoid building separate facilities. We need to develop locally based multi-purpose community facilities, providing a focus for collective community action.

Maximizing our access to and use of ordinary community facilities is inextricably linked with building alliances, identifying with and being identified by communities and our sense of accountability. It will be a reflection of the extent to which we are able to enter into dialogue and negotiate the definition of the problems that people face and the best solutions they put forward. Changing where we work demands that we dispose of the visible symbols of professional power in favour of meaningful, effective and enduring solutions to the true struggles that people face.

The Problems of Changing

The realignment of the relationship between us and those who use our skills will reflect a new alliance. We will seek to emphasize the things which unite us rather than divide us. However, within our new alliances we should not lose our responsibility to confront the attitudes, behaviour and problems of thinking that we see in the individuals or in the culture of the communities within which we work. Neither can our desire to promote the competence of each person allow us to deny the limitations and obstacles many people face in taking responsibility for themselves. We must not invest personal competence in those who do not possess it, or seek to impose change on people for whom to struggle is merely to stand still. Ours must be a 'reasoned faith' in the creative potential of each person, not a blind act of commitment to any ideology. We will continue to face individuals who desire and encourage us to offer a traditional response to their problems. But it is not adequate simply to assert that 'now that things are different', they are wrong to expect us to act in certain ways. We must accept responsibility to work from the point where each person starts, not from the point we think they should have reached. Trying to do what people want, whilst continually seeking to re-negotiate that want, is a mark of our new relationship. Our task is constantly to seek ways to help people transform their sense of the possible.

Our new alliances will bring new problems since the boundaries between those who use a given service and those who take a key responsibility to provide it, will be less clear. The alliances will open up opportunities for people to give support as well as receive it. There will be a new and more honest concept of 'well-being'. Consequently, we will need to develop a new code of 'ethics' which reflects and respects the different interests, roles and responsibilities of everyone participating in the service. A service within which there is a commitment to open nego-tiation as an instrument of therapeutic policy, will place con-siderable demands on those who are paid to provide and manage it. They will need support from those who manage them as employees. Further, they will need to develop effective ways to provide them with adequate care and encouragement. A new approach towards those who use our service demands a new approach towards each other. We will need to find ways to eliminate competitive, punishing and insensitive attitudes so deeply ingrained in all of us, and which feed from and into professional power.

The changes we need to make in our professional practice can only emerge through a change in our experience. As we begin to do things differently so we begin to experience the benefits of the changes we have made. This process of explo-ration is no different for us to the exploration for change which we seek to promote for the people who we try to support. What spurs us is a belief that things could be done better.

Making the changes necessary will not be easy. Many forces

are at work. Our own desire for power, status and acknowledgement will not simply disappear. The political, social and economic order will remain the same, at least in the foreseeable future. Throughout history there are few, if any, examples of those who hold power passing it willingly to those who are dispossessed. Whilst we can expose ourselves to the demands of those who use our services, we must never underestimate the power exerted over us by the views and opinions of our colleagues.

We must recognize the elements of our own thoughts and actions which mirror and perpetuate regressive community attitudes. We must acknowledge the principal source of our own motivation and concern. The structural 'needs' of a professional system of mental health care are such that they will continually conflict with the actual needs and wants of the people we seek to help. The politics of modern professionalized power is bounded by peer review. Modern heretics are those who support citizen competence and convert their profession into an understandable trade under the comprehensible command of citizens'.[6] To work 'with' rather than 'on' people, we will all need to be heretics!

Notes

1. P. Freire, *Pedagogy of the Oppressed*, Penguin 1972.
2. J. H. Galper, *The Politics of Social Services*, Prentice Hall 1977.
3. 'Ordinary Life Strategy', Derbyshire County Council Forward Look and Social Services Committee Minutes, 10 June 1982.
4. J. O'Brien, *Community Support Systems for People with Severe Mental Disabilities*, a background paper for the King's Fund Workshop, Planning Local Psychiatric Services, September 1983.
5. J. Chamberlin, *On Our Own: Patient-Controlled Alternatives to the Mental Health System*, Hawthorn Books 1978.
6. J. McKnight, 'Professionalized Service and Disabling Help' in I. Illich et al., *Disabling Professions*, Marion Boyars 1977.

15

The Independent Voice of Advocacy

DR BOB SANG

This chapter is based on my experience of the development of two forms of advocacy in the UK during the 1980s: self-advocacy and citizen advocacy. I will define the concepts, illustrate what they mean, and identify some tendencies which might endanger the growth of advocacy in this country. Finally, I will suggest some areas for action, hoping that this will stimulate wider involvement in an expanding movement.

The assumption behind my contribution is that traditional models of care, based on a partnership between professional service providers and voluntary self-help, are both limited and dangerous for people who have long-term needs; that the community care programmes and projects promoted by private, voluntary and public sector agencies, form a network of social control which could become as oppressive as the institutions they are designed to supplant; and that therefore it is no accident that people who use such services are now beginning to learn to assert themselves individually, in groups or networks, or with support from friends and independent advocates.

This assertiveness, which is reflected in the new advocacy movement, is an essential alternative to the Victorian values of self-help which have been promulgated as an integral part of contemporary community care services. In practice, self-help is code for low-cost and poor quality services – an abdication of responsibility by those who own and control the resources needed by thousands of people who are merely seeking a reasonable quality of life. Self-help means leave well alone, let families – especially women – take the responsibility, or leave people to fend for themselves in the private sector of greedy

190

landlords, shoddy bed and breakfast accommodation, and over-priced private rest and nursing homes.

Yet, within the care in the community arena there are many examples of good practice. Services which contribute to a good quality of life are sensitive to individual needs and wants and are genuinely people-centred – that is, managed and evaluated according to the expressed wishes of the service-users. In these situations the users have a real voice. This is essential if people do not directly own and control the resources needed to lead a decent life.

Self-help presumes that people make the best of what they are given. Advocacy helps them to assert their rights to much more than this.

Defining Terms

'Advocacy: active support especially of a cause.'
'Advocate : a person who upholds or defends a cause.
            : a person who intercedes on behalf of another.'
                                    – *Collins English Dictionary*,
                                      1980 edition.

These definitions are not complete, but they do broadly reflect most people's understanding of the non-legal meanings of advocacy and advocate. During the past ten or so years both words have been interpreted in a new more active way, especially in the so-called fields of 'mental handicap' and 'mental illness'. First in the US, then in Scandinavia, and now in the UK, more and more individuals, groups and organizations have become involved with or affected by the growth of an advocacy movement.

However, at a conference in 1984, William Bingley, MIND's Legal Director, issued a warning. He pointed out that because the word 'advocacy' was being used in a number of ways, some of them inappropriate, the concept was at risk of becoming debased, and of being taken over. 'At its loosest level professionals refer to advocacy as "raising a fuss" or "meeting clinical needs". This confused notion of equating advocacy with satisfying service needs ... leads, for instance, many social workers to define their role, as advocates on behalf of their clients.'[1] Heeding this warning, I will concern myself here with definitions of citizen advocacy and self-advocacy which are true to the spirit of the concept and I intend to challenge the claims made on behalf of two other forms: professional advocacy, and patients' advocacy.

Citizen advocacy occurs when an ordinary citizen develops a relationship with another person who risks social exclusion or other unfair treatment because of a handicap, illness or other, similar, disadvantage. As the relationship develops, the advocate chooses ways to understand, respond to, and represent the other person's interests as if they were the advocate's own.[2]

Self-advocacy occurs when an individual or group of individuals who use long-term public, private or voluntary services, begin to influence and eventually determine decisions which affect their lives. As they acquire and develop skills of communication, organization and self-determination, learned in an independent context, self-advocates achieve greater autonomy with regard to the effective representation of their interests as citizens.[3]

Both forms of advocacy emerged as a response to two fundamental characteristics of traditional services and their various institutions. The first is 'labelling'. A great number of organizational constitutions, articles of association, statutes, policies, plans, etc., are built round labels such as patient, resident, inmate, user, client, claimant, handicapped, disabled, mentally ill, disturbed, geriatric ... Affixed to selected individuals, these labels take away their specific identities. Instead they become defined and controlled by someone else.

I remember attending 'residents'' meetings at an old people's home on the south coast of England. All these meetings were run by management, usually the 'matron'. The agenda, timing, conduct, all reinforced the shared idea that these were, 'old people in care', so that the boundary round the lives of those who attended was confirmed and strengthened. How could anyone see elderly people in this situation as full citizens with rights, needs, wants and a future? Imagine living a life where you only had the power to discuss mealtimes, outings and 'no-smoking' rules!

But the majority of people who are labelled are not even accorded this dignity. Two particularly limiting and damaging labels are 'mentally handicapped' and 'mental patient'. Nearly all the self-advocacy groups I know are determined to secure the abolition of the term 'mental handicap', its derivatives and the commonly used alternatives such as 'subnormal', 'retarded', 'impaired'. Yet most of these people have to depend to a greater or lesser extent on services which use those labels in their policies and operational assumptions. Similarly, people labelled 'mental patients' have begun to organize themselves to confront the same contradiction.

The second potentially damaging characteristic is now clearly being exposed in the process of implementing the so-called care in the community policy – the cruel flaws, insensitivities, and impositions which are being perpetrated under the auspices of the humane idea of re-integrating people in ordinary neighbourhoods. I am talking about choice, or rather the fact that people have no choice.

In respect of self-advocacy the question of choice or no choice is emerging as a powerful component of the case against community care. On a recent visit to a small Sussex mental handicap hospital I was told by the hospital social worker, 'The patients here don't want to leave. They tell us so, because they know that moving will mean breaking up groups of friends who have been together for years.' This argument has been produced with increasing frequency in the media as the professional groups whose power-base lies in traditional institutions continue to assert their interests.

The horror stories of ex-hospital residents living in misery, isolation and despair in so-called community programmes run by private, public and voluntary service organizations, are building up to a cumulative picture of neglect and abuse on a massive scale.

When those remaining in hospitals and similar large institutions are questioned about future plans, it is little wonder that they are apprehensive. At no time had they been involved in the process which had led to the present situation. The practicalities of implementing community care policies have blatantly confirmed the almost total lack of power experienced by people who are labelled as 'ill' or 'handicapped'. It has also shown the dominance of professional and organizational control over their lives. They are now asked to react to a situation which is out of their control and threatens the few things they can call their own: a safe environment and the personal relationships they have been able to build up within the institution.

Asking someone's opinion when the choices open to them are virtually nil is a denial of self-advocacy. The purpose of my visit to the Sussex hospital was to talk with the residents about the possibilities of developing independent advocacy. I have not been invited back.

It is cruel irony that the opponents of care in the community now lay claim to self-advocacy in support of their case: 'Ask our residents ... They don't want to move.'

The crucial phrase in the definition of self-advocacy is 'learned in an independent context', which makes the concept either inexplicable or unacceptable to most service workers, especially managers. It means that self-advocates learn their skills and develop understanding independently from the system which dominates their situation. They gain a perspective on their lives which does not presume labelling and institutional rules. They become free to assert themselves and promote their interests as independent, equal citizens. Opportunities and risks can be evaluated in respect of responsibilities which are self-defined, not dominated or owned by 'responsible' service workers.

As self-advocates learn about themselves and the real choices open to them, they begin to make demands and ask questions which are not on the agenda set by those who have assumed full control. Let me provide one small, but significant example. My first self-advocacy conference was organized by people who attended day-centres in the London area.⁴ A sub-committee had independently set the agenda and provided the speakers. They had also invited some service managers, to listen and learn. One subject was the quality of food provided at work. The speaker spotted the manager of his local centre in the audience. Addressing him directly, he declared, 'I'm sorry, Mr Smith, the food people get at your place is rubbish. It is tasteless and un-healthy.' There was a great cheer from the audience, not because of the undoubted accuracy of the statement, but because, for the first time, self-advocates were putting quality of life issues on the agenda, on *their* terms and in *their* meeting.

Let us take this example a little further. The conference finished with a call to end the use of the term 'mental handicap'. How many people make a living out of this label? The resistance to change and the desire to subvert self-advocacy should not be underestimated. In my experience one of the most powerful people in any institutional service is the catering manager. The lives of such people are geared round deciding what and how others eat. If consumerism in respect of catering services is one consequence of self-advocacy, then prepare for a reaction from catering managers and the like. It is not just psychiatrists, social workers and nurses, who will be fighting to preserve the labels which give meaning to their job titles and their service organiz-ations ...

Citizen advocacy faces a similar challenge. It has emerged because so many people who use long-term services cannot, for one reason or another, speak for themselves in the way that self-advocates can. For instance, many people who have lived most of their lives in long-stay institutions have been denied the opportunity to develop the full range of communication skills; some lack confidence, others are actively suppressed and yet others lose the capacity to speak for themselves – older people, for example, who develop senile dementia.⁵

Citizen advocacy is not a service – a surrogate parenting or befriending agency designed to complement or support existing systems. It is an equal partnership between two people, one of whom is excluded from choices about life, and the other whose

196 Mental Health Care in Crisis

responsibility is primarily loyalty to and representation of their partner's interests.

Citizen advocates have entered into a wide and increasing variety of partnerships in this country. The early developments focused on people who were trapped in long-stay hospitals; but more recent community-based schemes are demonstrating how relevant citizen advocacy is in this context, to ensure a better future for people whose lives are regulated by the confusing panoply of community-based services.

The four key characteristics of a citizen advocacy scheme are its independence from formal service systems; its ability to support a large number of diverse partnerships without controlling them; the one-to-one sustained partnerships which characterize the advocacy relationship; and the diffuse informal network of people who value others as fellow citizens and refuse to acknowledge the labels and assumptions which dominate the statutory and voluntary service organizations. Citizen advocacy programmes offer a great deal of hope for all those people who are automatically excluded because they have no voice. They aim to provide that voice, and they do not intend to be controlled or limited by those who have held power by traditional right.[6]

The challenge facing all those who wish to promote and support the development of both self-advocacy and citizen advocacy is clear. It is a matter of finding ways to ensure that the thousands of people, who have a right to greatly enhanced self-determination and real autonomy, achieve a presence and a voice. The nature of this challenge can best be illustrated by looking at the 'People First' strategy, and by describing some of the people I met during my early work on advocacy and how the emerging movement began to touch on their lives.

People First

During the summer of 1981 I began to meet a wide variety of people who were interested in the relatively new concept of 'advocacy'. Earlier that year I had been appointed coordinator for the 'Advocacy Alliance'. The Alliance[7] was made up of five national charities, all of which were committed to improving the lives of people with 'mental handicaps'. At that time there was particular concern for the 45,000 people who lived all their lives in mental handicap hospitals.

My task[8] was to work in three such hospitals and introduce volunteer 'citizen advocates' to isolated residents who had no friends or relatives to advocate for them. I would like to describe the lives of some of the people I met, residents and advocates.

Colin[9]

When I met him, Colin was 20 years old. He had lived in a Surrey hospital for 16 years after his parents had been encouraged to put him into care because it was 'in both their interests'. He had been labelled severely mentally subnormal at a very early age. He was physically fit, very active, and articulate. He was the first person I met when I arrived. He approached me as I walked up the drive and enquired about my name and business before getting into a long list of complaints about life in general and his ward in particular.

To staff, Colin was trouble. His habits of going off on his own, attempting to make new acquaintances, walking into town, complaining, and taking up issues on behalf of other residents – all made him a difficult 'patient'. Yet after years of 'patient' treatment, Colin persisted.

Anyone who took the trouble to get to know him, soon recognized a sensitive, strong-willed and able young man. Someone who was, and is, prepared to advocate on his own and in ways which others found easy to put down to his 'sub-normality' or 'abnormal' 'disturbed' behaviour. While this labelling persisted, it was highly unlikely that Colin would be considered for any sort of life outside hospital, and this despite the fact that formally he was a voluntary patient. In fact his whole life was affected by the reality that he would have nowhere to go if he decided to leave. The hospital administrator told me that, for this reason alone, Colin and the great majority of other residents should be grateful for the home afforded them in the hospital!

Richard

Richard was Colin's closest friend. They clearly cared a great deal about each other and many of Colin's complaints were on Richard's behalf. Richard was also labelled 'subnormal'. In addition he was labelled 'non-verbal' and 'immobile', because he had a very limited vocabulary and depended on the use of a wheelchair.

They lived in the same, rather gloomy, ward with 20 or so men of similar ages. In common with the other residents Richard's personal belongings were kept in a locker by his bed and in a wardrobe opposite. Generally his daily life did not vary much: he attended the industrial training centre in the hospital grounds during the week, but spent a great deal of time in the ward. He was obviously bored and appeared to get depressed frequently. The monotony of his existence was broken by outings, organized by hard-pressed staff. Richard particularly enjoyed swimming, a liberating skill which he had developed over the years.

He was pleasant and humorous. Quick to smile, he was clearly very good-natured despite the dreary day-to-day quality of life he experienced. His friendship with Colin was very important, and through it I discovered that Richard was capable of a great deal more effective communication than was generally assumed. He could also be very mobile with help and was clearly determined to take advantage of any opportunity to get out and about.

Henry

I was introduced to Henry by his ward sister in a wing of what had once been known as 'The Institution for the Imbeciles of the Aristocracy'.[10] He had lived there for over 40 years – since his early twenties. He hardly spoke, always wore the same grey suit, and shuffled between the ward and the day-room, rarely venturing outside. I found it almost impossible to get to know him but from what I could gather, he hated going out and depended to a great extent on the routine that had been established on the ward and its adjacent day-room. He was labelled 'chronically institutionalized'.

I spent some time describing these three people first because I want to convey a sense of their individuality. Even in the case of Henry, whom I still hardly know, I can identify quite unique characteristics, needs, wants, desires and expectations. To plan major changes in the lives of these individuals without taking their wishes and opinions into account is inhumane. This applies to any community care initiative which might be considered for any or all three.

Secondly, if we ignore the labels that are attached to them largely for the convenience of the authorities, their existence is remarkably similar to that of others who are made dependent on institutional care – elderly people in private nursing homes, prisoners, children in care, physically disabled people in hostels and, of course, psychiatric patients or those who have left hospital and now have to depend on some form of residential or institutional support. They experience the same powerlessness, social exclusion, loss of identity and incredibly poor quality of life.

The most striking feature of their lives is the 'institutional thought structure' which surrounds them. In common with the 'users', 'consumers', 'residents', 'clients', etc., of all other welfare services, they are the objects of a set of processes which are devaluing and invalidating. Certainly, they have no hope of ownership or control of the services which encapsulate their lives. In this respect, the voluntary, private and public sectors are all the same: real power and final authority rests with their bureaucratic elites.

Colin, Richard and Henry now have advocates who have been involved with them for over four years . Colin's and Richard's advocates are actively pursuing a home for them to live in together outside the hospital. Every step, every decision, is worked out collectively, with Colin's and Richard's preferences and choices driving the whole process along. It is taking a long time. Not because resources are not available, but because the attitudes and values of those who control the resources stand in the way of positive change. They are not prepared to let 'their children' run 'their services'! These problems have a long history – from the moment when Richard's advocate pointed out that he did not want anyone, especially staff, going into his locker. Then came the battle for a better wheelchair; the fight to get access to the local swimming pool; Colin's refusal to take drugs; achieving the right to mobility allowance; buying their own clothes; making and keeping friends from 'outside'. Not typical for young men in their twenties in the 1980s.

Henry now chooses to go out regularly with his advocate. He is rapidly gaining a wide experience of the world that he left 40 years ago. With that experience he is developing an understanding of the real choices which are available to him. This 'chronically institutionalized' man is openly contemplating moving out of the hospital.

So who are these advocates? Supermen and superwomen, well-versed in welfare rights law with the skills of barristers and professional negotiators?

Mary[11] is Colin's advocate. Her husband is a school teacher and they have two school-age children. Her part-time work brought her into contact with the local voluntary network and, by a circuitous route, she contacted me. She met Colin at a social event we organized. They seemed to hit it off from the start and, as their relationship developed, the advocacy programme provided her with some training, advice and expertise, and a lot of support during tough times.

Joan has partnered up with Richard. She has a full-time job and her children have all left home. Her husband gets involved in advocacy too. For example, he drove the car to the local pool when Richard wanted to go swimming one weekend. He then drove them round to the local town hall when the pool attendant would not admit them: 'Disabled only on Thursday afternoon.' He drove them back when they had seen the Director of Leisure and Recreation, having achieved the necessary change in policy.

Bill retired from business a few years ago. He is about the same age as Henry and they have a good mutual understanding.

Henry let everyone know what he thought of Bill when, just before Bill's third visit, he went and waited for him in the car park. Another of his labels was 'agoraphobic'!

This is really all that needs to be said about advocates. They are ordinary citizens who made a choice to become involved on the basis of mutual trust and loyalty. They are not paid to be there. They are not professionals. They are not 'voluntary workers'. They value others as they would wish to be valued. They are resilient and determined. They ignore labels and other prejudice. There are now about 150 such citizen advocates in various schemes in the UK.[12]

Threats to Advocacy

It is easy to imagine that any advocacy scheme, self- or citizen advocacy, will experience opposition, ranging from determined attempts to stifle it at birth, to persistent undermining and controlling by groups and individuals who work for the 'clients' best interests'. There is no escape from this. Too much is at stake. The vast range of services that have built up and which have now become more diffuse, diversified and overlapping, with the advent of community care have just created more opportunities for professionals and administrators to export their model of rules and strictures which controls the lives of thousands of individuals. The 'top-down model of care' does not presume a truly effective voice from those who have to use the service organizations and their resources.

Anyone who gets involved in advocacy is aware of all this and knows that the trick is to ignore this morass and get on with getting things done. Make your own rules and agendas; they are almost certain to be clearer, simpler and more achievable than the decisions which emanate from the health and welfare bureaucracies.

The real threat to advocacy is that it is being undermined from within and in its very earliest stages. The two aspects to this threat are professional involvement and institutional control.

Earlier on I stressed the crucial importance of the independent development of advocacy. Independence means, in particular, autonomy in respect of any service organization or professional interest. Yet, everywhere I read and hear of new initiatives in community care which include advocacy in their charters and terms of reference. Let me quote three examples:

- A charity for 'the mentally handicapped' which is funding a self-advocacy group run by a social worker.
- A joint-financed residential scheme for 'ex-hospital patients' which states, 'We shall ensure that every one of our residents who wants one will be found an advocate.'
- A day-centre which has an 'advocacy session' every fortnight.

All over the country people are writing advocacy into their policy documents. Professionals are being trained in advocacy principles and skills. Funding is even being set aside to promote advocacy 'in the best interests of the service users'. Thanks, but no thanks! The consequence of all this well-intentioned activity is a 'bandwagon' effect which must suit senior managers and planners very well. It is flavour of the month when it comes to scoring points in the 'progressive and humane awareness' league table.

I must confess I used to think that this might be one way forward. Get the system on our side and we might get somewhere. How naive! By all means let people know what's going on. Let professionals share in an understanding of what it means to enable individuals to find a real voice of their own. But also let them learn that it is not their business how this voice emerges, who organizes it and how it expresses itself.

Professional involvement is not just inappropriate, it puts any advocacy scheme at risk. Unfortunately, this simple message runs contrary to the vocational ideology of 'professional advocacy'. How often do we hear the message: 'Nurses are the patients' advocates' or 'Social workers are their clients' advocates'? Indeed, most professional training includes an element of advocacy these days – quite rightly. But the vocational assumptions, which underpin the various professions and their approved training schemes, ignore the unresolvable conflicts of interest and values that exist between service users and service providers. Professional advocacy is a limited tool which is seen at its best when it is directed by the service user, not the service provider. Yet, all too often, professional advocacy is the only form of advocacy available, especially for those who cannot speak for themselves: people who are trapped in long-term residential and domiciliary situations.

This point is best illustrated by an examination of the issue of institutional control. The early attempts to initiate self-advocacy and citizen advocacy in the UK have been bedevilled by this. Many of the early self-advocacy groups developed in day-centres or adult training centres for 'the mentally handicapped' (the label already implies the problems).[13] Time to meet, agendas, facilities and support were often controlled and directed by 'management'. Advocacy groups may be very successful for a while. But, if they become too autonomous, if they begin to address difficult issues, then many of the resources upon which they depend start to be withdrawn. This is why the 'People First' network was started — to meet in non-service buildings, to raise its own funding, and to use non-professional advisers. Again, independence is the key.

Now there is also the emergence of 'patients' advocacy' in psychiatric services. Generally stimulated and organized by professionals, it involves people who share the same label 'patient' and attend or use the same service institution. Because patients' advocacy activities are clearly so much more positive than those generally experienced by, for example, psychiatric hospital residents, this form of advocacy has been acclaimed as a major step forward. In fact, it is a major defeat for independent advocacy.

Anti-psychiatry professionals have leapt aboard the band-wagon, conveniently forgetting the fundamental contradictions which exist between them and their patients. Institutional facilities and organizational resources are giving the patients their say and 'they' are even allowed to influence management decisions. This is often seen as supportive of community care because it 'improves social and other relevant skills'. From beginning to end patients' advocacy is run to suit the interests of institutions which are being forced to change in the face of new policies. The fact that it appears progressive is a reflection of the power of the controlling forces which exist within psychiatric services and which come openly into play as soon as 'clinical judgement' and other professional rights are challenged.

Initiating Independent Advocacy

Begin with people first. Identify a few friends you trust. Get together and discuss some of the ideas you like in this publication and the references. Meet because you are friends and citizens, not because you share a label, or because you want to help someone who is labelled. Remember that the objectives of independent advocacy are clear and positive: the full rights of citizenship and social integration on terms acceptable to the individual.

People who become involved with self-advocacy need to learn to work as a mutually supportive and openly democratic group. This takes time and a lot of learning. When important issues emerge which entail challenging others, think carefully about tactics. Advocacy does not necessarily mean confrontation. It does not exclude it either. Start with small successes and identify the 'no strings' support that you might need. Keep the network growing!

Citizen advocacy poses another sort of challenge. Self-advocates often know people who need citizen advocacy: listen to them. Citizen advocacy does not have to be a scheme or a programme. It can just be a loose group or set of people who get to know others, who are at risk of social exclusion. Maybe you know of a woman in a private nursing home who is never visited and who cannot speak for herself? You may also know someone who is prepared to spend some time getting to know her and her wants and needs. It will not be easy; but unless she, and other people in similar situations, are found a voice they will continue to be excluded.

But, if the people who get involved with citizen advocacy are independent, if they are persistent and flexible, and if they learn to support each other, then their networks will grow and interconnect, become visible and develop a strength of their own.

Notes

1. William Bingley, 'Advocacy – Setting the Scene' in *Advocacy and People with Long-term Disabilities*, Kings Fund Reports 1985.
2. This definition largely belongs to John O'Brien. See Bob Sang and John O'Brien, *Advocacy*, Kings Fund 1984, Project Paper No. 51, p. 33.
3. This is my definition, based on experience and observation.
4. Their members belong to the 'People First' network of the London area.
5. For a detailed discussion of the relevance of advocacy to such people, see Bob Sang, 'Advocacy and People with Dementia', Appendix I in *Living Well into Old Age*, Kings Fund Project Paper 1986, No. 63.
6. Amanda Forrest, *Citizen Advocacy – Including the Excluded*, obtainable from Sheffield Advocacy Project, 14–18 West Bar Green, Sheffield.
7. The Advocacy Alliance was founded by MIND, MENCAP, The Spastics Society, The Leonard Cheshire Foundation and One-to-One.
8. This work is fully written up in Sang and O'Brien, *Advocacy*.
9. The names I use here are fictitious, but the account is based on real people and their recent experiences.
10. Normansfield in Teddington, Middlesex.
11. Again the names are fictitious to preserve confidentiality.
12. This approximation derives from the eight schemes which I have been able to identify. New ones are beginning to emerge in an encouragingly unstructured way.
13. For this history see Paul Williams and Bonnie Shoultz, *We Can Speak For Ourselves*, Souvenir Press 1982.

16

The Self-Advocacy Movement in the UK

PETER CAMPBELL

In November 1985 MIND's National Conference was called 'From Patients to People'. It was the first time a national conference in the mental health field had privileged the views of service users. Users gave presentations to the full conference, spoke from the platform, led and co-led workshops and sub-plenary groups. It was an event of some symbolic significance. Around the same time the concept of self-advocacy was emerging – a phrase which in essence is tautological and which seems certainly to have been the invention of professionals, or at least of professional journals. In the space of 18 months or so, it had taken over to such an extent that people in user groups – people like myself – began to accept that what we were doing was indeed 'self-advocacy', and to talk about ourselves and others as self-advocates. This chapter is not an attempt to analyze a concrete phenomenon, to pin it dead on the board, but rather to describe from an insider's viewpoint, a new and developing activism among service users, to give an impression of what is going on, what may be behind it and more crucially what it may mean in the future.

A major and somewhat contradictory feature of self-advocacy is the important role mental health workers play in it. Although groups are not dependent on the active involvement of workers, the current position self-advocacy holds would not have been achieved without the stimulus and support of a small but significant number of concerned and energetic workers. It is significant that there are only two self-advocacy groups in Britain that claim to be user-only – Campaign Against Psychiatric Oppression (CAPO) and Sagacity in Community Care (SICC). The majority of existing groups are alliances of users and workers with a smaller element of 'carers', each alliance weighted in a different way. The problems inherent in such alliances and the implications they may have as activism increases across the country, are difficulties self-advocacy has yet to resolve.

In a more general sense the position of the mental health worker and the psychiatric professional has been crucial. One of the major impulses leading to self-advocacy in the mid-1980s as opposed to frustration in the 1970s, has been the obvious concern about the future of psychiatry among many who work within it. In short, psychiatry seems to be in greater disarray now than at any time since 1945. The dominance of the psychiatrist within the system is now clearly under challenge. The old Victorian asylums, the playing fields of old style psychiatry, are closing down. On different pitches the game may well be played to different rules. Mental health workers faced with the imminence of care in the community have been looking around with concern for different ways. This groundswell of unease has not gone unnoticed by users. In the context of our traditional powerlessness the fact that workers start glancing in our direction is the primary symptom, the only symptom, that we need to embark on our own diagnosis.

There is a long tradition of protest against psychiatry. This should not be surprising. In Britain psychiatric treatment is supported by compulsion, a fact which has implications for all who are cared for within the system, whether detained or voluntary patients, and which may have some bearing on the numbers who emerge from an ostensibly caring process feeling that they have been punished. For whatever reasons there is a smaller community of interest between carer and cared-for within psychiatry than almost any other branch of medicine. Thomas Szasz has spoken of psychiatry as an area of religion and philosophy rather than of science. Many medical students doubt whether psychiatry has a scientific basis. In the light of these uncertainties it cannot be extraordinary that many recipients of this doubtful expertise claim the right to voice their own concerns. One of the elements integral to current self-advocacy is this fundamental and long-established protest out of powerlessness. There are direct links between groups of the 1970s anti-psychiatry movement, such as the Mental Patients' Union (MPU) and Prompt, and groups now campaigning, such as CAPO and the British Network for Alternatives to Psychiatry (BNAP).

I believe it is important to realize that self-advocacy groups do reflect a real mood, both within society and within the society of the so-called mentally ill. Since 1945, oppressed minorities within Western industrial society have taken huge and positive steps to confront their devalued status. Black power, women's liberation, gay liberation have all become significant social movements. The so-called mentally ill may be mad but we're certainly not stupid. Though a continually de-valued class we have nevertheless changed considerably over the last 30 years. It is one thing to treat people with indignity, locked away beyond society for years or decades. To treat people with indignity and allow them, indeed encourage them, to share society with you as protected and mistrusted lap-dogs is something else altogether. As a result of 'open-door' policies and chemotherapy, users now believe they are part of the community; indeed, they have no general reason to doubt that they are. Yet in reality although they are invited to the party they are forced to sit out on most of the dances. I was diagnosed psychotic at 17. I have been a service user for 20 years. Yet at no time have I been beyond the community for more than a year consecutively. I am part of the community. I have always been part of the community. To be treated as a second-class human being in these circumstances is a bitter cut. The strength of self-advocacy is that it is founded on a changing self-image among service users. It is a self-image which historical and social realities now confirm.

One of the characteristics of current self-advocacy is its diversity. Compared to the anti-psychiatry movement of the late 1960s and the 1970s, self-advocacy in the 1980s seems to have a broader base and to be more rooted in the realities of the local, as opposed to the national or global, situation. It is possible to question how much impact the ideas and sophisticated arguments of R. D. Laing and David Cooper had at ground level. While remaining open to the criticism that as activists we do not truly represent the spectrum of service users, most of those involved in self-advocacy groups are aware of the realities and are working towards concrete and realizable goals. As a result it is difficult to talk in terms of 'national platforms' or even of a 'self-advocacy movement' in too close a sense.

There are now over a dozen groups in this country speaking and acting for themselves in the area of mental health. London has the preponderance of groups as might be expected. Five boroughs north of the river – Ealing, Barnet, Camden, Islington and Hackney have self-advocacy groups. But outside of London there are also large and flourishing groups: Glasgow, Chesterfield, Nottingham and Bristol. In other cities like Southampton there are the beginnings of groups run by users. Based in London but with a national focus there are also the two campaigning organizations, which I have mentioned before, CAPO and BNAP. Finally, acting as an umbrella organization, campaigning and fund-raising towards a national conference of service users and their allies, is Survivors Speak Out, which was established in November 1985 following the MIND conference in London. When viewed against the background of the previous five or six years the achievements of these last two or three begin to look quite significant.

The degree of unity between the existing groups is conditioned by a number of factors. In the first place it is not clear to what extent they are all asking and working for the same things. In the second the approach of different groups is influenced by their differing structures.

The voice of the service user as expressed in self-advocacy groups encompasses a broad range. At one end there are those who are voicing openly abolitionist views, who would not wish to work with psychiatry and psychiatrists but only to replace them and the oppressive system they command. At the other end there are those who, whilst speaking up against their status and role in society, appear only to be seeking improved services provided by a more enlightened state system. In between lie a number of related positions, some of which imply that the only way to improve services or change the system adequately is to have elements of user-run services within it while others suggest more strongly that user consultation in planning and monitoring of services might be adequate to secure the necessary change. While there does appear to be broad agreement on the goals, the means of reaching them, and in particular the priorities in terms of immediate practical action, seem to be open to discussion. To some degree this is inevitable. It would be wrong to under-estimate the broad sweep of service users' concerns. On a micro-cosmic level self-advocacy is addressing itself to the psychiatric system. On a macrocosmic level self-advocates in mental health are challenging the whole position of a class of people within' society. The psychiatric system is a target, a major target indeed, but within a wider scheme. At this stage, with groups so small and with so many avenues available and opening to pressure, it may well be a sign of vitality that there is no unified voice. It is possible that many voices with a unity of feeling will prove to be the most powerful weapon the service user can present.

In broad terms there are three main types of group. First, the national campaign groups: CAPO and BNAP. Though based in London they address themselves to the whole of Britain, do not concentrate on local matters, but campaign on major issues affecting the whole psychiatric system such as the abolition of ECT, no compulsory element in psychiatry, the provision of adequate facilities for withdrawal from major tranquillizers. At present they are not significantly involved in service provision. They have no premises of their own and exist on minimal funding. They are limited in size – as are all self-advocacy groups – but extremely active in certain areas where they are now being noticed increasingly.

The second category might be called the locality-based group. Camden Mental Health Consortium, Barnet Action for Mental Health, Hackney Mental Health Action Group are some London examples. This type of group, quite often set up with initial involvement by community health councils, concentrates on its local area and on the problems of the psychiatric system as expressed in the local services. While they may share the concerns of the first category they are as likely to work on specific problems in day-care provision in their area as to take on broader campaigning issues. In summer 1986, Consortium, the first user group to seek involvement in the planning process, produced a report on provisions within Camden based on a questionnaire to members. This was presented to the relevant authorities and has led to a recognition of Consortium's claim to a role in future consultative processes. At present this group is predominantly involved in campaigning and pressure group activities. It has made a conscious decision not to get involved in service provision. Whether any of the other locality-based groups will remain solely campaigning critics of the system is not yet clear. The gap between the hoped-for and the actuality, the tardiness of current providers, may well propel such groups into the role of alternative suppliers of much needed facilities. Nevertheless at this point they remain largely without premises, existing on small funds.

The third category is made up of groups which are connected to existing service provisions or which are themselves supplying significant services. 'Link' attached to Glasgow Association for Mental Health and 'Contact' at the Tontine Road Centre in Chesterfield are examples of the former, while Bristol Women and Mental Health – an umbrella covering a number of services for women in Bristol – is the notable example of the latter. These groups differ in various ways from the other two categories. They are certainly more stable both in terms of structure and funding and because the users involved are in more regular contact. Their range of activities are wider, their organization more complicated. To some extent they escape the feeling of impermanence, of imminent dissolution, which hangs around many of the impecunious campaigning groups. To some degree they bring a welcome solidity to self-advocacy.

Finally mention must be made of the Nottingham Patient Council Support Group (NPCSG) which is establishing the idea of patients' councils within psychiatric hospitals along lines inspired by the example of the Patients' Councils in Holland.

Their work with a particular set of ideas in a particular context is unique in Britain, highly important, and could prove to be one of the most significant developments of the mid-1980s in terms of confronting user powerlessness.

The evidence above indicates there is considerable activity in the area of self-advocacy. There is some cause to believe that it will not all be ephemeral. Although most groups are numerically small – I do not think that more than 400 people at the most are directly and actively involved in Britain at present – they are shifting some of the traditional obstacles. For many years the existence of MIND, the National Association for Mental Health, as a liberal, professional and comparatively well-funded pressure group, forced independent user groups onto the fringe – the loony left. It was unnecessary for the establishment to address users directly. This is altering. On the one hand it is clear that MIND and other agencies are now entertaining groups and individuals that ten years ago they would have ushered out through a side-door. On the other hand it is becoming apparent that existing groups now have an influence and positive existence in their own right. Doors that were once closed are being left ajar. The present dimensions of self-advocacy do not encourage easy marginalization.

Even so most groups face an uncertain future. They suffer problems common to all small ill-funded groups. They work in a field where the potential to initiate constructive change is only just becoming apparent. To some extent all existing self-advocacy groups have taken on the role of pioneers and suffer the joys and insecurities of such a position. They must run quite hard in order to maintain their position.

Money is one problem. Although a small campaigning group operating in a defined locality can be effective on quite restricted funds, the size of a group and the extent of its influence is limited by lack of resources. At present funding bodies appear either to be ignorant of self-advocacy groups or to assume that they are a spontaneous and natural phenomenon which does not demand active support. As a result, groups appear to be cutting each others' throats, applying in competition to the few known sources of funding. The possibility of groups evolving from a campaigning to a service provision role seems remote in such a climate. The degree to which self-advocacy groups are dependent on the established system of authorities' official bodies and charitable agencies is a crucial unresolved issue.

For it is not only the absence of money which restricts, but also the terms and conditions which the acquisition of funding, of official approval, may come to impose. The danger of co-option is very real. It is quite conceivable that funding bodies will be more willing to fund the provision of 'tea and sympathy' facilities run by service users than to support genuine alternative services. At the same time current evidence suggests that the DHSS and other bodies are intent on creating – from the top downwards – some element of user representation on planning and management groups. This is not self-advocacy. But the danger exists either that self-advocates will be sucked upwards into this new and alien mechanism or that the impulse towards self-advocacy will be ignored while bureaucracy seeks a more manageable input into its machine. Despite the achievements of the last few years no one should forget who is the shepherd and who is the giant.

Nevertheless the show is definitely on the road. There are rough edges and the lighting effects may be a bit ropey. But the sense of optimism, of enjoyment, is unmistakable and there is no doubt in my mind that the potential of self-advocacy is huge. All I can say in conclusion is that there has been a sea-change among service users and that it is a continuing pleasure and privilege to be part of it. The next five years could be good ones for the future mental health of the nation.

Index

214